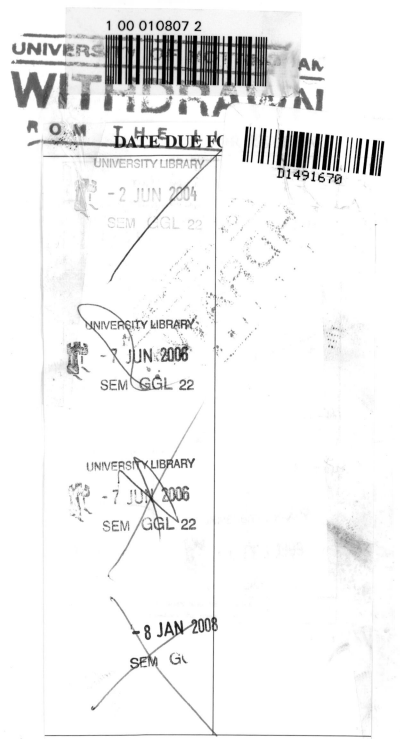
This book may be recalled before the above date.

Clinical Trials
an introduction

SECOND EDITION

U NOTT

Clinical Trials
an introduction

SECOND EDITION

Ann Raven

with a Foreword by Frank Wells

Radcliffe Medical Press, Oxford and New York

© 1993 Radcliffe Medical Press Ltd
15 Kings Meadow, Ferry, Hinksey Road, Oxford OX2 0DP

This title was previously published as Consider it Pure Joy
and distributed by A Raven Publication, Cambridge.

British Library Cataloguing in Publication Data

A catalogue record for this book is available from the British
Library.

ISBN 1 85775 035 7

Typeset by Advance Typesetting Ltd, Oxfordshire
Printed and bound in Great Britain

Contents

Foreword

The discipline of clinical research is tough. No professional, or indeed any other person, involved in the conduct of such research should be under any illusion about this. Standards must be upheld, and any deviation from what has been agreed must be effectively, although discreetly, dealt with. It therefore makes it so much easier to do this if one has a basic understanding of what clinical research is all about, why newer and better medicines are needed, and how they are developed.

Guidelines on many aspects of clinical research currently abound. Some of them are on the conduct of research, others are on relationships between the various persons who are involved in research projects and yet others are on the ethical standards which should apply to any clinical trial. Some guidelines assume the status of rules or law, and so a working knowledge of what is required by regulation is essential for those involved. However, such guidelines tend to be turgid and read as official documents, whereas this book is intended to be strictly practical and easily read. Indeed, Ann Raven succeeds in presenting a great deal of valuable information and providing many answers to the questions which might be raised by someone joining the discipline of clinical research for the first time—whilst also providing a sound commentary on the basic principles of clinical research which more experienced persons in the field will find of great value.

Ann Raven has written in a style which enables the written word to flow off the page, and that makes its assimilation easy. Readers will find that they remember what they have read, and will truly enjoy tackling the trials which lie ahead.

DR FRANK WELLS
Director, Department of
Medicine, Science and Technology, ABPI

Preface

Successful clinical drug development relies on the united endeavours of a multitude of people. Some are rather visible: doctors and patients and the senior medical executives of the pharmaceutical industry. There is a plethora of sophisticated textbooks for physicians and scientists, and complex guidelines abound. This book is written for the unsung heroes, whose names seldom appear on publications and who may never visit the research centres, but whose role is vital. There is now a vast army of administrative and technical staff who work in the offices, libraries, laboratories, data management departments and pharmacies and who support this complex process.

For all those who are new to the industry and for whom the jargon of clinical trials is something of a mystery, I have tried to present a brief introduction to the process and to explain and define some of the expressions employed.

The first edition was produced primarily for my own support staff in a large clinical trials department, but I was encouraged to publish it. It has since been used as the basis of training and induction courses in the pharmaceutical industry in Europe and the USA, to provide career guidance for those aspiring to join the industry and also in medical schools. I am delighted that sales have more than justified a wider audience and hope that this second edition proves useful.

Ann Raven
September 1993

Acknowledgements

I would like to acknowledge the aid and encouragement of many friends and colleagues, both in industry and academia, especially those who have made helpful suggestions for this new edition. I am grateful for the patience and skills of Juliet Corfield who prepared the manuscript.

About the Author

Ann Raven is a consultant in Trials Management and Training, advising companies on management and clinical trials systems and training programmes for their medical department staff. She joined the pharmaceutical industry in 1976 and has since worked as a CRA and subsequently as Head of Trials Management for DAR Ltd, a contract research organization. From 1985–89 she was the Education Officer for ACRPI. In this role she instigated and organized the Introduction to Clinical Trials Course and was instrumental in setting up the University of Wales postgraduate Diploma in Clinical Science. For three years she was a Tutor in Clinical Research at Cardiff. In 1989 she initiated (jointly) the UK CRA Training Forum. When managing a large department of CRAs and their support staff, she implemented her belief that secretaries, data managers and information scientists should be offered training in parallel to CRAs, in a comprehensive ongoing training programme.

Drug Development

How are new drugs discovered?

Drugs have been in use for thousands of years and come from many and various sources. They include plant and animal extracts, antibiotics from micro-organisms and an assortment of synthetic chemical compounds. Today, there are about 1000 medicinal compounds in common use, most of which have been developed from a few dozen 'prototypes'.

Plant extracts have lost much of their popularity in this country since the majority are much more toxic than their synthetic equivalents and only a few new drugs have been discovered from this source in the last 50 years.

A significant advance in drug research was the discovery of organ extracts. For example, the lives of millions of diabetic patients were saved following the isolation of insulin in 1921.

The value of controlled experiments with animals was established in the early 1890s and, for at least 50 years it has become usual for drug development to follow a pattern. Most new drugs are modelled on existing prototype drugs, natural (animal, plant or mineral) products or hormones. A chemical compound is produced and tested on animals; structural changes are then made to the molecule to influence the biological activity until the desired effects are seen. Pharmacologists have developed sophisticated screening tests to help them recognize promising new drugs. These tests usually involve inducing the target disease or symptoms in an animal species. The development of such **animal models** has done much to improve the understanding of disease process as well as treatment. When such a compound emerges from screening the chemists often produce **analogues** — compounds with a very similar chemical structure. These also enter the screening programme in the hope that one or more of the series will be both safe and effective.

This rational approach has been greatly enhanced by the combination of chance and judgement known as 'serendipity'. Many of the most successful drugs used today were identified as a result of chance observations during the search for something quite different.

What happens before drugs are tested on people?

In the 20th century, people have come to expect and demand safety and an almost complete lack of toxicity (literally, poisoning) for the ever-increasing variety of drugs they consume. Whilst some drugs (particularly plant extracts) produce adverse effects immediately, many appear to be perfectly safe until they are taken over a long period of time. Therefore, once a prospective new drug has demonstrated a specific and interesting activity in the animal model, it must be subjected to a battery of toxicity tests in animals before it can be given to people.

In Europe it is normal practice to perform acute and chronic toxicity testing in a rodent species, eg rat/mouse, and a non-rodent, eg rabbit or dog. In the USA three different species must be tested. Trained technicians observe the effects on the animals, first using single doses of the test drug and later repeated doses. Both sexes of animals of various ages are studied. Following the test period those animals which are sacrificed are examined minutely.

The objectives of these tests are to establish what adverse effects or toxicity occurs and at what dose. For example, some drugs will cause liver damage, but only at high doses.

Rigorous guidelines for these tests are provided by regulatory authorities relating to the species and numbers of animals, duration of testing and doses to be employed — relative to the intended use in humans.

In addition to normal toxicity testing, the effects of a new drug on fertility (reproductive toxicity) and on the fetus must be established (teratology tests). Long-term safety and carcinogenicity tests in animals are conducted once the drug is approved for testing in patients.

Whilst animal toxicity tests are being conducted, many other activities take place which are also important for the drug development process, *see* Figure 1. Production chemists will be developing manufacturing methods, others will be exploring different pharmaceutical formulations and conducting tests to find out how stable the drug is, at room temperature and in other conditions. More detailed pharmacology testing will be underway to establish not only likely benefits in man but also potential side-effects. Later, studies will be conducted to investigate whether the new drug interacts with other drugs when taken at the same time. Metabolic tests which show how the drug is absorbed, distributed around the body and then broken down and excreted, will be conducted in animals. Pharmacokinetic studies, which measure the rate at which the drugs are absorbed and enter the blood and how long it stays there, are conducted in animals and later in human volunteers. Results from these studies may provide a useful prediction of future efficacy and safety.

About the time that the drug is first tested on humans, the manufacturing process is scaled up and commercial-sized batches of the newly formulated drug begin production.

It is estimated that only one in 10 000 compounds, selected for further development after initial screening, progresses to a product licence in man. Most compounds are rejected in the acute toxicity testing process.

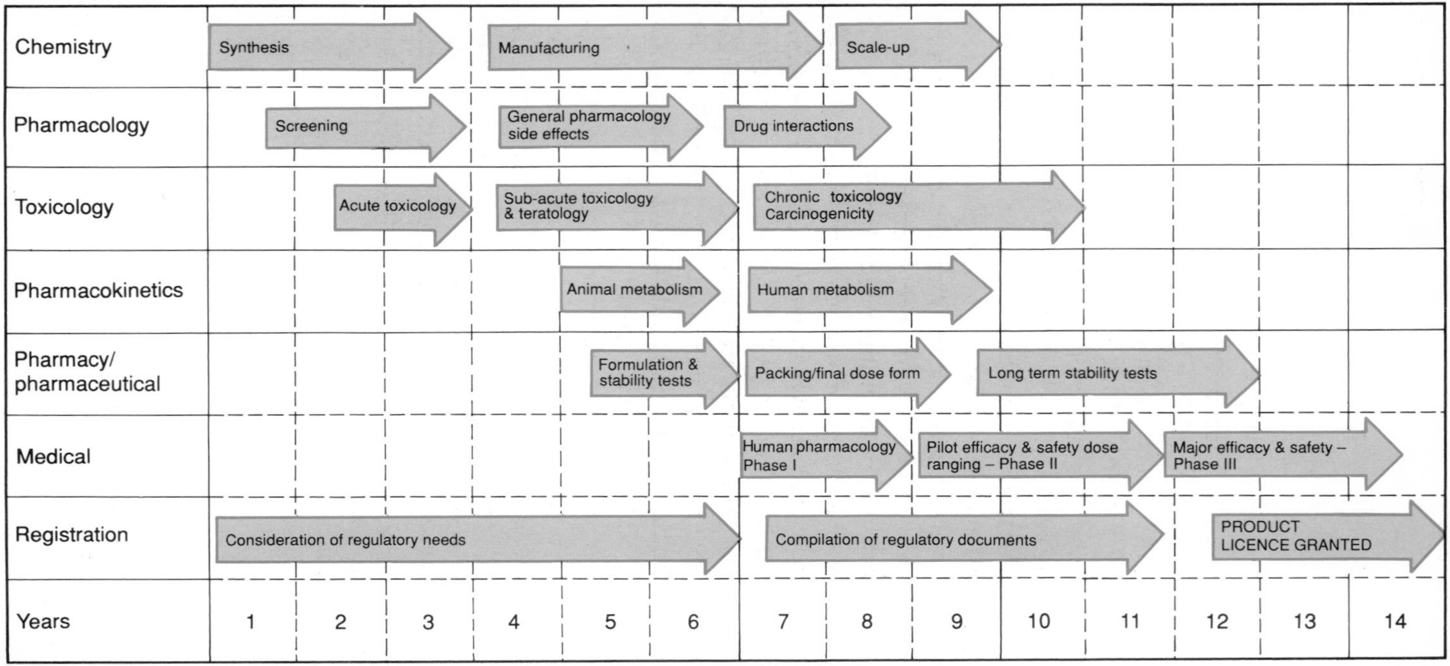

Figure 1: A simplified scheme of new drug development

The table/chart presents the following information across categories and years (1–14):

Chemistry	Synthesis; Manufacturing; Scale-up
Pharmacology	Screening; General pharmacology side effects; Drug interactions
Toxicology	Acute toxicology; Sub-acute toxicology & teratology; Chronic toxicology / Carcinogenicity
Pharmacokinetics	Animal metabolism; Human metabolism
Pharmacy/ pharmaceutical	Formulation & stability tests; Packing/final dose form; Long term stability tests
Medical	Human pharmacology Phase I; Pilot efficacy & safety dose ranging – Phase II; Major efficacy & safety – Phase III
Registration	Consideration of regulatory needs; Compilation of regulatory documents; PRODUCT LICENCE GRANTED
Years	1 2 3 4 5 6 7 8 9 10 11 12 13 14

Why are human volunteer trials performed?

For most new drugs, it is considered preferable to conduct tests in healthy human volunteers before exposing 'sick' patients to them. Unlike the USA, at present it is not necessary to obtain permission for these trials from the regulatory authority in the UK. However, these trials, like those in patients, must be approved by an independent ethics committee.

Volunteer trials, also called Phase I trials, are conducted in hospitals or commercial human pharmacology units, where specialist medical attention could be immediately available if a serious adverse event occurred. The objective is to establish how the human body handles the new drug and what toxic effects, if any, are experienced. First, single doses are given, in slowly increasing quantities and then, if all appears to be well, repeated doses are given to different individuals. These trials are invariably placebo-controlled and involve only very limited numbers of healthy volunteers. They are monitored with extreme care throughout the trial. Volunteers are often pharmaceutical company employees or medical students — traditionally, healthy young men who are paid for their involvement. Recent legislation also now demands that new drugs intended for an elderly population must also be tested in 'healthy' elderly volunteers. There are some drugs, such as chemotherapy agents used in cancer treatment, which could not be tested ethically in healthy volunteers. These special categories of drugs are tested only on selected 'patient volunteers', in hospitals.

How are drugs tested on patients?

Following Phase I trials in non-patient volunteers, clinical trials in patients are divided into a number of further phases.

Phase II describes the first patient trials: these will be very carefully controlled trials aiming to give an idea of efficacy, which dose is optimal and some preliminary information on safety. This Phase will usually involve only a few hundred patients. Some of the trials are likely to be placebo-controlled and frequently they are conducted in hospitals. If the results from Phase II are sufficiently promising and all the rest of the drug development process is progressing smoothly the drug company may decide to embark on the more expensive Phase III.

Phase III trials are the major efficacy and safety trials, often involving thousands of patients. Most of these trials will be conducted under the same conditions as would prevail once the drug was marketed, but with closer monitoring. Many Phase III trials are conducted therefore in general practice. This Phase will include comparative trials with other marketed treatments and also placebo-controlled trials. The results of the Phase III trials will be required before an application for a product licence can be submitted.

Phase IV trials are those performed after a drug has received a product licence and is marketed. Many questions may remain unanswered, such as effectiveness and safety in children or the elderly. Large post-marketing surveillance (PMS) studies are now often conducted on new drugs to identify rare adverse events. These also serve to establish the general usefulness of a new drug used in normal clinical practice in a significant number of patients.

Named patient treatment is a mechanism wherein an unlicensed drug can be supplied to a doctor for the treatment of a particular (named) patient. Pharmaceutical companies are usually sympathetic to these requests, particularly where no alternative therapy is available, but the patient must be carefully monitored and a report submitted to the company.

Regulation of Drug Research

Who makes the rules?

Before new drugs can be administered to patients, approval must, by law, be sought from the national regulatory authority.

In most countries, a panel of scientists employed by the national government reviews the available data and decides whether to grant permission for specific clinical trials to proceed. In some countries the company or individual researcher simply has to notify the government of their intentions.

In the USA, the regulatory authority is known as the Food and Drug Administration (FDA) and clinical trials must be registered with this body via a Notice of Claimed Investigational Exemption for a New Drug (IND) which lays down the purpose and conduct of each trial.

In the UK, since the Medicines Act 1968, there has been a comprehensive system of drug licensing which is handled by the Department of Health. The licensing authority can issue product licences, manufacturer's licences and Clinical Trial Certificates (CTCs). There are a number of advisory committees consisting of independent experts including the Committee on Safety of Medicines (CSM) which advise on safety, efficacy and quality of new medicines. A sub-committee of the CSM investigates adverse event reports. Clinical trials in patients should be covered by a clinical trial certificate or a Product Licence (PL), but since 1981 most trials have been conducted under the Clinical Trial Certificate Exemption (CTX) scheme. Under this scheme, only a summary of the pre-clinical data and the trial protocol are submitted to the Medicines Control Agency (MCA). If the expert assessors find the data acceptable they will grant a CTX within 35 days. If the CTX submission is rejected, the company must apply for a full CTC which may take many months.

The EC Commission has set up a Committee for Proprietary Medicinal Products (CPMP) in Brussels which is developing a system of mutual recognition between member states to reduce the duplication of evaluation of PL data. There are plans for a central EC regulatory agency and, meanwhile, multi-state Product Licence Applications (PLA) have begun to be employed. However, the complex process of harmonization of the national drug regulatory authorities is proceeding slowly.

How are the drugs assessed?

Teams of expert assessors which include pharmacists, toxicologists, pharmacologists and clinicians review all the pre-clinical data and decide if the drug is safe to be given to patients — before a CTC, CTX or IND equivalent is granted.

During the clinical trial, annual progress reports are usually submitted and all serious adverse events must be reported. When clinical development is completed a huge dossier containing all the pre-clinical, efficacy and safety data, together with a number of expert reports, is compiled and submitted for a PL. The review process may take between six and 30 months for a PLA, depending on the country and type of drug involved.

What about ethics?

In addition to a scientific review of information on the drug, clinical trials are subject to various ethical controls.

The Declaration of Helsinki is almost universally accepted as the standard code of ethics on human experimentation. Whilst accepting that progress in medicine requires experimenting on humans, this document describes basic ethical principles including the requirement to obtain informed consent from each subject and an obligation to submit the protocol to an independent ethics committee for comment and guidance. A copy can be found in Appendix 7, page 81.

Most hospitals and all health authorities in the UK have an ethics committee which consists primarily, but not exclusively, of medical staff. In some countries there are regional and even national ethics committees. Their composition and conduct is governed by slightly different guidelines in each country. In the UK there are several sets, the most well-established being published by the Royal College of Physicians. Usually ethics committees meet up to ten times a year, although some still review protocols by post. The main objectives are to review trial protocols to ensure firstly that the trial is well-designed and justified from the data available, and secondly that the risk to patients is minimal. Local ethics committees will also consider whether the facilities or staffing levels at the hospital or clinic are adequate for the proposed trial.

Since ethics is not an absolute subject, there is much controversy about what should be permitted. For example, the use of placebos in severely-ill patients will be unacceptable to many. Conducting studies on children, the mentally ill or pregnant women also present particular ethical problems.

Very occasionally a pharmaceutical company will request permission to conduct a trial for marketing reasons. If the science is inadequate, these are rarely justifiable, and may be rejected by an ethics committee. In the UK, if any ethics committee rejects proposals for a clinical trial, the regulatory authority should be notified. In many European countries, regulatory authorities consider the opinion of the ethics committee before giving their permission to conduct the trial.

What is informed consent?

Patients who are invited to participate in clinical trials should be provided with adequate information about the trial before making their decision. Usually the doctor will explain the reason for the trial, briefly what is known about the test drug(s) and what measurements and procedures are involved. Absolute confidentiality in the trial report should be assured, although permission may be sought for the pharmaceutical company medical department staff to review the patients' notes. The patients should be told that involvement is purely voluntary and that they are free to change their mind and withdraw from the trial at any time. Normally the patient is also given this information in writing and should be allowed sufficient time to consider and, if necessary, ask any questions.

Patients should not be offered any inducement to participate in a clinical trial and may not be paid, although travelling expenses may be offered, if appropriate, and trial drugs should be provided free of charge.

If the patients understand the implications and agree to participate, they are usually asked to sign a consent form, which is kept in their hospital/GP notes.

Good Clinical Practice

3

What is Good Clinical Practice?

When the American FDA coined the phrase 'Good Clinical Practice' (GCP) they might have predicted that it would cause widespread offence, for surely Good Clinical Practice is our expectation of any medical practitioner? Originally, GCP was a set of proposals prepared and published in 1977 for the guidance of investigators and pharmaceutical companies undertaking clinical trials in the USA. They were prepared as a response to anxieties about the quality and reliability of some of the research data submitted to the regulatory authorities.

Although not popular even in the country of origin, the main tenets of the GCP proposals were that clinical trials should be good science, verifiable, monitored, well-documented and comply with high ethical standards. The basic principles have been accepted now by USA, Japanese and European pharmaceutical companies. GCP guidelines have already been prepared by the Association of the British Pharmaceutical Industry (ABPI) in the UK and by French, German and Nordic authorities. In 1991, an EEC working party published European GCP guidelines and these are now being widely implemented. A copy can be found in Appendix 8, page 85.

The subjects encompassed by the GCP guidelines are:

▼ the selection of investigators
▼ protocol content
▼ ethics committees and informed consent

▼ trial monitoring, data validation and source data verification

▼ adverse event reporting

▼ drug accountability

▼ data handling, use of computers and statistical analysis

▼ content of trial reports

▼ standard operating procedures (SOPs) and quality assurance

▼ archiving of case record forms (CRFs) and trial documentation.

They are primarily organized under headings of 'sponsor' (pharmaceutical company) or 'investigator' responsibilities. One common theme throughout can be simplified as 'write down your procedures, then document what you do and be prepared for inspection'.

Why is GCP necessary?

Developing drugs is an expensive and lengthy business (it may cost £100 million over more than 12 years for one drug), and it is undesirable to have to repeat the process in different parts of the world. It is therefore a good idea to ensure that the research data is acceptable to all the regulatory authorities. Since the USA is the largest single market for pharmaceuticals, most pharmaceutical companies wish to be successful there. The FDA will review clinical trial data only if it is conducted to GCP standards. Certainly the EEC GCP guidelines are culturally more acceptable to Europeans and less rigid in some areas. Their implementation is doubtless improving the quality of clinical trials sponsored by the drug industry.

What difference does GCP make?

As companies implement the GCP guidelines they are realizing that there is a high price to pay for increasing standards — more staff are needed, each co-ordinating fewer trials with greater care. Clinical trials need not take any longer — and with more care about trial design and selecting investigators they could proceed more quickly — but there is about a three-fold increase in the number of monitoring and secretarial support staff needed. In addition, SOPs must be written and a GCP Quality Assurance department established to conduct internal audits.

Not all staff will take kindly to following SOPs or being audited, especially if they have been doing the job for years(!), so training and compliance programmes need to be set up. More documents means more filing and storage can be a significant problem in some departments.

Finally, an important difference should be the confidence with which everyone can view the results of a clinical trial. The satisfaction of passing a stringent audit should not be underestimated!

Clinical Investigators

Who are investigators?

On first hearing this expression you may think that this term refers to a kind of medical CIA! In fact, it is simply what the drug industry calls those who 'investigate' new treatments in patients. Invariably they are doctors who are sufficiently senior to have their own patients — in the UK this means a general practitioner (GP) in the community or a consultant or more senior academic in a hospital. The senior person at any 'investigating' centre is termed the 'principal investigator' and he or she may delegate much of the work to co-investigators, often junior doctors or research nurses and pharmacists. The principal investigator, however, retains legal responsibility. Sometimes in trials conducted in many centres (multicentre trials) there is an overall principal or co-ordinating investigator who may have a major role in designing the study, recommending other clinical investigators, interpreting and publishing the results.

Where do investigators work?

Investigators may work anywhere providing they have access to a suitable group of patients and facilities for examining and assessing them. Early studies with a new drug are normally conducted by investigators based in an academic university department of a teaching hospital. Larger studies are more frequently done in district general hospitals — with either in- or out-patients, depending on the drug. Recently, in the UK, there has been an increased emphasis on training in general practice — both of doctors and nurses. As a result of this and also improved facilities in health centres, many more drug trials are now being conducted in the community. Health care systems vary considerably throughout Europe, but everywhere the trend is towards an increase in Phase III trials in the primary health care setting.

How do you find investigators?

Finding the ideal investigator to conduct a trial is one of the greatest challenges for clinical trial staff. You need to find someone with considerable medical skill, commitment to research, good facilities, willingness to fill in endless forms and finally, access to lots of patients who trust him/her and who will consent to enrol in clinical trials. The most obvious approach is to speak to previous contacts and friends in the specialty and ask their advice. Anyone publishing a paper in one of the specialist medical journals is likely to be quite motivated in that field, so a literature search can be fruitful (doctors who start trials but never finish them do not usually publish). Some investigators are identified at conferences — every specialty has its own society and meetings. The Medical Register includes all British registered doctors together with their qualifications. In addition, the Medical Directory, published annually, theoretically lists all British doctors alphabetically and also all hospitals by region. This two volume tome is a mine of useful information. Each doctor entry gives details of training, qualifications, memberships of societies, major publications, current and previous jobs. Hospital entries list all consultants by department. In addition, doctors are listed by town and village if you prefer to make a geographical selection. In the back pages you will find addresses and staff details of universities and postgraduate institutes. (It is not comprehensive, however, and occasionally someone's name is missing; this does not mean they have been 'struck off', it could be that they simply did not return the entry form in time or are only very recently qualified.) Most European countries have a similar register of medical practitioners.

Once suitable potential investigators have been identified, the drug company CRA (or medical adviser) will approach them to discuss: (1) whether they wish to participate in a clinical trial, and (2) whether they and their facilities are acceptable to the company. Not every qualified clinician is a successful investigator and in recent years many companies and health authorities have had cause to compile a blacklist of doctors who have demonstrated an inability to conduct clinical trials correctly.

How is an investigator addressed?

Like many professionals, doctors are rightly proud of their qualifications and therefore it is important to understand them and their job titles. A newly qualified British doctor has to complete a pre-registration year as a houseman or house officer. Later he or she is promoted to senior house officer (SHO). The next step is registrar in a specialty and two or three years later, senior registrar (SR). For many doctors the final step is promotion from SR to consultant and, once appointed, consultants rarely move. In university (teaching) hospitals, a lecturer is equivalent to an SR and a senior lecturer to a consultant. The head of an academic department may be a reader or a professor. On occasions eminent doctors have what they call a 'personal chair', that is, one which was created solely for them and will not be passed on. On retirement, these are termed Emeritus professors.

At registrar level, hospital doctors usually study for postgraduate qualifications from the appropriate Royal

College, to obtain, for example, membership of the Royal College of Physicians (MRCP, UK), Fellowship of the Royal College of Surgeons (FRCS) and possibly a research doctorate (MD) in their chosen specialty. A surgeon in the UK, who is an FRCS, is entitled to be called Mr (Miss or Mrs) instead of Dr and obstetricians in England and Wales also follow this practice. In Scotland, obstetricians consider this to be Sassenach nonsense, and retain Dr throughout! GPs in the UK are likely to have completed a three-year post-graduate vocational training to become accredited and they can also take membership exams to join the Royal College of General Practitioners (RCGP). However well-qualified, only partners in a GP practice may have their own list of patients.

The abbreviations and usage of common UK medical qualifications are included in Appendix 4, page 75 and Appendix 5, page 77.

Why become an investigator?

What motivates a doctor to add to their already hectic and demanding lifestyle by getting involved in clinical trials? Providing there is definite motivation, perhaps the exact reason is unimportant, but it should be understood that it is rarely primarily for personal gain, either financial or in prestige. Drug trials for pharmaceutical registration are infinitely more tedious in respect of form-filling than any research a doctor might design himself, and sometimes the individual doctor has no input into drug company trial design at all. Consultants often consider trials to be good training or discipline for their juniors. The research grants may help to fund badly-needed equipment, an extra pair of hands in the clinic or even a trip to an academic meeting in an exotic location! Usually there is a genuine concern to be contributing to the search for better treatments. A complicated trial may assist with team-building and improve staff morale in, for example, psychogeriatric wards. Some doctors are quite simply flattered to be approached to undertake research with a new and potentially exciting drug.

What is the investigator's role?

Without clinical investigators the drug industry could not develop drugs. The industry is, therefore, completely dependent on a group of professionals who are not accountable to them and who are ultimately the only market. Investigators are central to the whole concept of clinical trials. They have an important role in trial design, case record form (CRF) design, obtaining ethics committee approval, selecting patients, obtaining consent and treating and assessing patients in a trial. They also bear legal and moral responsibility for each individual patient's welfare. They can be expected to supervise (or delegate) the dispensing of and accounting for drug supplies. Investigators must complete and retain complex .documentation for the pharmaceutical company and report any undesirable effects in trial patients. The industry expects investigators not only to participate in clinical trials, but to adhere to schedules, recruitment rates and protocols which the sponsor dictates. It all sounds extremely burdensome, but amazingly enough the majority of investigators are pleased to interact with the pharmaceutical industry and are invariably and genuinely welcoming to clinical trials staff (CRAs and others) who visit them regularly. For many industry people working in clinical trials, the great attraction of the job is the interest and pleasure in collaborating with clinical investigators.

Trial Design and Protocols

What is trial design?

Every clinical trial is an experiment which aims to improve knowledge about a new treatment for patients. The question to be answered may be quite simply 'does it work?' or 'is it safe?'. Usually doctors want to be more precise than this, so it is common to ask 'is this new drug better than the old one, either in terms of treating the disease better or quicker, or in terms of the same benefits but with fewer side-effects?'. There are many different ways to test the risks and benefits of new treatments; the trick is to choose the design which gives you an answer to the question as quickly as possible and involves the minimum number of patients in the experiment. The design of the trial is a description of the way patients will be studied, in terms of selection, treatment and assessment.

The most usual design in drug trials is the **group comparison**, in which patients are randomly allocated to either of two or more different groups which receive different treatments and the responses of each group are then compared.

Alternatively, you can compare the effect of one treatment after another on the same individual, and these are called **cross-over trials**. These trials only involve half the number of patients overall, but each patient is studied for twice as long as in a group comparison.

Sensible researchers often do a pilot study before the clinical trial begins. As the name suggests, this is a mini-study involving limited numbers of patients. The objective is usually to ensure that the chosen design, patient selection and trial procedures are feasible.

Who is the designer?

Clinical trials may be designed by a medical adviser or CRA within a drug company medical department. Alternatively, the design may be proposed by a doctor or even a medical group who might then approach the drug company asking for supplies of a new drug treatment.

How are trials designed?

When pharmaceutical company staff are involved, they are usually not specialists in every aspect of trial design, so they have to spend some time asking for advice and generally finding out how to proceed.

Questions which need to be asked are as follows.

▼ What are the objectives?
▼ Which disease should be treated (this is sometimes called the indication for treatment)?
▼ What sort of patients might benefit (eg age, sex, duration and severity of illness)?
▼ How do you measure the disease?
▼ How can you best measure response to treatments?
▼ How many patients do you need to study?
▼ Where are the patients normally treated (eg general practice, hospital in-patient departments, specialist clinics)?
▼ What safety tests should you employ?
▼ How long should you (1) treat and (2) study patients?

▼ How much of the test drug should you give (eg dose, frequency and duration)?

▼ What should you compare it with?

▼ What do the regulatory authorities permit/require?

From this list alone you can see that a lot of specialist advice from doctors and nurses in the appropriate disease area, potential investigators, pharmacists, technical and laboratory staff, statisticians and regulatory affairs personnel will be required.

The designer must obtain all this information, collate it and then draft a trial protocol. The protocol should be agreed upon by all the contributors and formally approved by the pharmaceutical company, investigator, ethics committee and regulatory authority.

How are trials controlled?

Clinical trials are often described as 'controlled'. This is where groups of patients are managed in an identical way apart from the test treatment they receive. If factors such as exercise, diet, medications other than the trial drug, etc could influence the progress of the disease, they should, if possible, be the same for all patients in a trial. Often the control group receive a well-established (reference) drug for comparison. This would be called an 'active' control. But controlled studies do not always involve a comparison with another drug. One group of patients may be untreated; some patients fare very well without drug treatment, possibly due to the disease being of short duration or even due to the effect of seeing their doctor or nurse more regularly and receiving extra attention, which is inevitably the case when patients are involved in clinical trials. This is particularly common in elderly, perhaps isolated, patients, and in those with psychiatric problems. Another 'inactive' control is placebo 'treatment'.

What is a placebo?

This is an inactive substance (often chalk or lactose) which is made up to match the test drug, either as a tablet, capsule, injection or even as an inhaled or cream preparation. Considerable improvements are often seen in patients 'treated' with placebos. This is known as placebo response and can be a major problem to pharmaceutical companies who usually have to prove that a new drug is better than a placebo. Sometimes one-third, or even half of the patients will respond adequately to placebos. Unfortunately, you cannot predict which patients will do well on placebo treatment. Also, in some conditions it can be very difficult or even unethical to employ a placebo control. Doctors must exercise particular care in monitoring patients in these trials.

How many patients should be involved in a trial?

To have a complete understanding of the usefulness of a new drug, it might be ideal to give it to all the people suffering from the disease or condition which the drug is intended to treat. This would mean treating the whole patient population. Of course, this is unlikely to be either feasible or even desirable. So a sample of the population has to be selected which is representative. If it is a good sample, the results of the trial should be relevant and applicable to the population. It is important, both ethically and scientifically, for the sample to be big enough to detect a true difference between two treatments that is of clinical importance. The measure of this ability to detect a real difference is called the power of the trial. This can be used to calculate a suitable sample size if you can establish in advance at difference between two treatments would be clinically significant.

How are patients allocated to each treatment within the trial?

Clinical trials, like any experiment, need to avoid bias. Bias can be introduced by the doctor, who may have a preference for one treatment, or by the individual patient or even by the choice of design itself which could favour one treatment. The first way to avoid bias is to randomize patients onto one or other treatment so neither the doctor nor the patient can predict which treatments each patient will receive. In practice, the drugs are packed and numbered according to a random list and patients are then given the next available numbered pack when they enter the trial.

Whilst most trials proceed as suitable patients turn up at the clinic, sometimes it is possible to collect a significant number of patients who all start the trial on the same day. These groups of patients are called cohorts (the implication of military precision is probably over-optimistic!).

Occasionally, it may be useful to evaluate patients' suitability for a trial over a few days or weeks. Chronic diseases such as asthma, angina and epilepsy cannot be assessed adequately on one occasion, so the patients may be entered into a run-in phase while they, for example, complete a diary card and learn about the measurement techniques prior to allocation to trial drug(s). Sometimes this time is used to reduce and stop other drug therapies which would interfere with the trial, and this is commonly termed a washout.

What is a blind trial?

Trials where everyone is aware of the treatment received by the patient are called 'open'. Examples of these would be trials of surgical devices, contraceptive devices or any comparison where treatment cannot be matched, like radiotherapy compared with drug therapy in cancer patients.

Many clinical trials, however, test drugs which can be matched and the doctor and/or the patient are unaware which treatment is being given. These are called blind studies, either single blind or double blind. Blinding is another way to minimize bias.

It is quite difficult to match different drugs so that they not only look and taste identical, but can also be given with the same frequency. Sometimes it is impossible to match the drugs, eg a drug given by injection and one in tablet form, but you can still keep doctor and patients 'blind' by making up dummy injections and dummy tablets, each patient receiving either a dummy injection and an active tablet, or a dummy tablet and an active injection, according to a random allocation. This approach, not surprisingly, is called double dummy

What is a protocol?

The protocol is the name given to the design document. It is quite complex and may take several months to develop and finalize. There are fairly strict guidelines (eg ABPI, EEC GCP, FDA) which dictate what they should contain. The following is simply a list of headings.

▼ Introduction and rationale.
▼ Aims/objectives.
▼ Trial design.
▼ Schedule.
▼ Patient selection criteria.
▼ Trial medication details.
▼ Procedures
       allocation to treatment
       informed consent
       clinical assessments
       laboratory assessments
       adverse events and emergencies
       concomitant medication
       trial documentation
       patient withdrawals.

▼ Monitoring and audit procedures.
▼ Trial commencement and termination.
▼ Statistical analysis.
▼ Reporting and publication.
▼ Ethical and legal issues.
▼ References.
▼ Appendices (including summary).

A good protocol should be clearly indexed, not least because many different parties need to refer to it. It must be clear and understandable to doctors and nurses conducting the trial, ethics committees and the regulatory authority giving approval, the CRA co-ordinating the project, pharmacists, statisticians and regulatory affairs personnel, strategy, planning and, possibly, marketing personnel from the company. The protocol may form the basis of contracts (between companies and sub-contractors, for example, laboratories and clinicians) so it is undesirable to change it once approved. Protocols are also central to clinical trial regulation (as explained in Chapter 2) and any amendment results in a repetition of the approval process which is both time-consuming and expensive.

Case Record Forms

6

What is a case record form?

At the end of a clinical trial, after possibly several years of work, the only tangible product is a collection of pieces of paper called case record or case report forms (CRFs). These are the forms on which all the information and results of the clinical trial are recorded. They are designed to match the protocol, be filled in by the investigator, checked by the CRA and the results put onto a computer for analysis. A common source of confusion is that CRF is also used as an abbreviation for case record *folder* which is a bound 'book' of individual forms, sufficient for one trial patient.

How are CRFs designed and produced?

Many CRFs are designed by the CRA responsible for a trial, although larger companies may have a separate department which both designs and produces them. It is a real skill to structure the questionnaire or form so that it not only collects all the necessary information but is easy to complete, unambiguous and convenient for entering the data into a computer. Those who, like the author, struggle with tax return forms, will be familiar with the frustrations of filling in a complex form. Consider how much worse it must be to complete a ten page CRF whilst maintaining a caring consultation with a severely-ill patient. There is a great temptation to design the CRF primarily to suit the person who checks it and/or enters the data onto the computer. However, if the form does not accommodate the doctor or patient completing it, the poor quality of information collected and the amount of errors and omissions can compromise the entire project. With the advent of word processing and desk-top publishing packages, form design has become easier to do in-house. Many CRAs and their secretaries can now produce print-ready proofs. Again, a word of warning: however smart they look, it is important to show draft copies to the investigators and ask them to try the CRFs with a few patients and scribble on them with red ink. Doctors, like other mortals, thoroughly enjoy correcting and editing your script!

These days, CRFs are fairly standardized and they usually include the following elements:

▼ information and consent forms ⎫ beginning
▽ patient selection checklist ⎬ of trial
▼ patient medical history ⎭ only

▼ medication records ⎫ repeated
▼ clinical and laboratory assessments ⎬ at each
▼ adverse event forms ⎭ visit

▼ end of study/withdrawal forms.

Whilst the majority of the information is usually recorded by the investigator, many trials also include patient self-assessment forms or diary cards and special care is needed to ensure these are easy to complete.

Usually each form is identified by a number designating each investigator or centre, the patient number and the date of assessment; each will also be signed by the investigator.

Once they have been drafted, commented on by investigators and data entry staff/statisticians and redrafted, CRFs are printed on NCR (no carbon required) paper and bound into books or folders. Often these are colour-coded and have smart outer boards printed with flow charts and aide-mémoires for the investigator and dividers between each visit. They are also usually perforated for easy removal of individual sheets from the folder. A secretary with a good eye for colour co-ordination and design may contribute much to this process. If the printing, collating and binding is done in-house, it is a considerable labour of love, although satisfying (particularly for a small study!) and needs careful quality control.

What happens to completed CRFs?

Once the patient's involvement in the study is over and the doctor has completed the CRF, it is usually checked on site by the CRA and then brought back to the office. The investigator is given one copy and the originals are forwarded to the data management or biometrics department. The information on the CRFs will then be extracted by data-entry staff and entered onto a specially-designed database ready for analysis. Usually the computer carries out checks on the data for consistency and against the protocol. It is usual for the CRA to retain a spare copy in case data management personnel identify any queries or omissions. These should be answered or corrected by the investigator. Once the whole study is completed, the original CRFs will be archived by a drug company for 15 years, or the lifetime of the product. The investigator must retain a register of the identification of trial patients for 15 years after trial completion.

Trial Supplies

7

What do you need for a trial?

In addition to a protocol and CRFs you need sufficient quantities of the drugs to be investigated to treat all the trial patients for the agreed period. It may be necessary to provide equipment for measuring the disease process and taking biological samples (blood, urine, swabs, skin samples etc). Also, a considerable number of documents for each investigator need to be prepared.

How are drug supplies obtained?

Once drugs are marketed, obtaining supplies is relatively simple. With the appropriate authority they can be ordered from pharmaceutical wholesalers or direct from the manufacturing companies. When the drug is still in development, it is usually produced in smaller quantities and might only be available from a research pharmacy. If the drug is to be compared with another and they are to be 'blind' it will be necessary to obtain unmarked tablets or pure drug material from the other manufacturer. Often, the CRA is able to simply send an appropriate requisition form to their clinical trials pharmacist who then orders drugs in bulk, packs them in bottles or blister packs and labels and packages them. In a smaller company you may have the challenge of preparing the randomization list, ordering, packing and labelling your own supplies. This must all be supervised by a pharmacist in a suitable room. The labelling of trial drugs is most important and there are strict guidelines for each country and variations for some hospitals and certain classes of drugs. Once they arrive, the drug supplies must be kept in a secure (usually cool) room until dispatched to investigator centres. Careful records must be kept of stock and transport arrangements.

What medical equipment is needed?

It is quite common for the pharmaceutical company sponsoring a drug trial to provide the necessary equipment. This may be because it is desirable to standardize equipment or measurement techniques or simply because an otherwise suitable investigating centre lacks the appropriate technology. Often it is a centrifuge (used for spinning blood samples) or a freezer for storing blood or urine samples. The former are often available from contract (central) pathology laboratories or specialist rental firms who provide a delivery, maintenance and collection service. If your trial involves electrocardiogram (ECG) or blood pressure measurements, several companies offer a service providing a variety of machines (including 24-hour heart monitors), interpreting the results and providing brief reports on each patient.

If medical equipment is recalled and re-issued, it is sensible to arrange for a full service and a check on calibration before despatch. You may get involved in purchasing and distributing large and sophisticated equipment for some trials. Often the technician or junior doctor who will use it lacks training and the responsibility for arranging suitable instruction may fall on the CRA and their colleagues.

Where shall we do the blood tests?

Since it is now common to undertake multi-centre studies, pharmaceutical companies increasingly choose to employ a central pathology laboratory to perform all routine haematology or biochemistry safety tests on samples from every investigating centre. This makes the results easier to analyse because every local laboratory has slightly different methods and **normal ranges**. These central or contract laboratories usually produce, on request, individualized test request forms (for inclusion in the CRF) and sample collection kits (syringes, needles, swabs, storage tubes and post-paid containers). The samples are posted direct to the laboratory who send the analysis reports to the investigators and CRA within about 24 hours. Most investigators find this approach very convenient and hospital out-patients are saved a long wait for the hospital laboratory.

What documents do you need?

When the study is started or 'initiated' a number of documents should be provided by the drug company.

▼ Indemnity statements (from the company to the doctor). These explain that the company will take responsibility for any drug-related problems providing the doctor keeps to the agreed protocol.
▼ CV form. The doctor must provide a CV or complete a form describing his qualifications, experience, current position and workload.
▼ Investigator agreement or statement. In this document the doctor agrees to fulfil all his responsibilities and adhere to the protocol, enrolling and treating patients within an agreed schedule.

▼ Financial agreement/letter. This contains the terms and details of the money to be paid to the doctor or his hospital/research fund (often per patient).

▼ Protocol. Often this has a page for final signatures.

▼ Declaration of Helsinki.

▼ Compensation guidelines. (ABPI (1991) in the UK) These explain procedures and conditions for payment of compensation to patients.

▼ CRFs and informed consent forms. These will include information sheets for patients to read and consent forms for them to sign.

▼ Adverse (drug) event reporting forms.

▼ Trial register. A list for recording patient's names and hospital numbers against their trial numbers.

▼ Dispensing list/drug accountability form. Forms for recording dates when patients receive and return their trial drug supplies.

▼ Sealed code envelopes. Individual numbered envelopes which identify patients' treatments in a blind trial (for emergencies).

▼ Investigator brochure. A booklet concerning all previous work reported with the test drug from the chemistry and pharmacy and animal work to early human trials.

▼ Investigator responsibilities list or GCP guidelines or explanatory booklet.

▼ Copy of regulatory approval to conduct the trial.

▼ Laboratory normal ranges (if a central laboratory is being employed).

All these will be available or generated in-house and are usually collated in an investigator trial file so they can be explained, assimilated and stored conveniently. The investigator must add to this long list a letter of approval from his ethics committee before the trial can start.

How do you account for trial supplies?

Trial drugs and documents are both important and valuable and, therefore, care must be taken not only in storing and transporting them but also in documenting the process. The amount of drug issued should equal the amount the patient takes plus unused drug returned. This is called drug accountability. Someone must ensure that exact records are kept at both the investigating site (receipt, dispensing and returns) and the drug company. There may be a separate department of pharmacists working on this full-time — or a locked cool room and forms to complete within the trials department. Unused and date-expired drug supplies may need to be destroyed, in which case a certificate of incineration should be obtained. It is sensible to deliver and collect trial supplies by hand and, failing this, by a reliable courier service — the normal postal system is not adequate. Some of the documents have legal significance so it may be useful to log them in and out. Finally, trial supplies may require considerable amounts of secure storage space, ideally with convenient access for the trials department staff, since most supplies need to be personalized.

Clinical Research Associates

Who becomes a CRA?

Clinical Research Associates (CRAs), also called clinical trial co-ordinators/scientists/officers/executives or **monitors** in different companies, are usually graduates with a background in a biological science, eg zoology, pharmacology, biochemistry, pharmacy or **physiology**. They should be able to communicate well, both verbally and in writing. They need to have very good personal skills — people should enjoy meeting them and they should be persuasive. Very often this means they have considerable personal confidence and are quite mature and interesting people. Obviously they must be bright and presentable because they are dealing with sophisticated professionals (doctors and medical scientists, as well as pharmacologists, etc). Over the past ten years, the job has become more controlled, so CRAs also need to be rather obsessive in terms of checking CRFs and meticulous in formally reporting, for example, any adverse events which patients might experience.

Fifteen years ago monitoring clinical trials for a drug company was a natural progression for a medical representative. These independent individuals were familiar with the medical profession and their company's range of drugs and were also used to travelling extensively. These days it is unusual for a representative to become a CRA unless the company wants to do Phase IV (marketed drug) trials with a predominantly 'field-based' team of monitors.

It is now more usual for companies to employ scientists with research or laboratory experience. Often a PhD is a requirement, certainly for some of the senior posts or for early development phases where there is more 'science' involved. A few companies will employ non-graduate nurses and technicians. These people, as junior CRAs, will probably need further qualifications for any promotion. On occasions, secretaries working for a medical department have been sponsored to do a part-time degree and become CRAs. Most CRAs have an office in the medical or clinical research department of a company. Some CRAs work from home, either on a freelance basis or for one company. This arrangement obviously reduces travel and modern technology has improved the quality of communications between the medical department and these field-based staff. In some European countries it is common to employ medically qualified CRAs.

What do CRAs do?

The CRA is primarily a co-ordinator and 'enabler' of drug trials. Twenty years ago most of this work was done by a company medical adviser who had many other responsibilities. Now there are about 2000 CRAs in the UK alone. As research into drugs becomes more regulated and therefore expensive, pharmaceutical companies cannot afford to develop drugs slowly or with poor quality data. The industry believes that a trial will be better organized, run more to schedule and produce better data if it is co-ordinated by CRAs. The industry has been proved right. Doctors' principal responsibility is to care for individual patients, not to conduct trials with complicated paperwork and numerous extra patient assessments.

So the CRA may be involved in designing the study and preparing the protocol and CRFs. They will usually select suitable investigators and organize all the trial supplies and any necessary training/instruction on trial procedures at the investigating centre. They will assist the investigator in obtaining ethics committee approval and liaise with their regulatory colleagues who will apply for permission to conduct the trial. They will arrange any necessary laboratory tests and liaise with pharmacies about storing and dispensing the trial drugs. Most CRAs also negotiate and supervise payment for all aspects of the clinical trial and arrange any investigator 'contract' which their company imposes.

Once the trial is under way, the CRA visits the investigator on a regular basis, to help with any problem that may hinder the smooth progress of the trial and to ensure patients are being treated according to the protocol. This will mean checking every patient's details against the selection criteria and comparing their recorded assessments with agreed procedures. The CRA needs to find out if all safety tests have been carried out and the results considered carefully; that proper informed consent is obtained from every patient and that the correct amount of drug is administered. This may all seem to suggest that doctors are not competent — this is not so! However, protocols are very complex documents and it is very easy to overlook, for example, that the patient is taking another drug which might interact with the new (test) drug or perhaps has a history of disease which does not comply with the exact terms of the protocol, eg an old peptic ulcer which might exclude them from involvement with a new drug for rheumatism, many of which can cause stomach problems. The manufacturer or developer of a new drug is given permission to do only carefully controlled studies and is responsible for ensuring that unsuitable patients are not exposed to a new and unlicensed drug.

The CRA must also make sure that the trial runs to schedule — and this is possibly the greatest challenge. If you need to study 100 patients to draw conclusions from a trial it is no good at all having 27 at the end of the period, however well-controlled or high-quality the data.

The CRA's lifestyle is varied and usually hectic. Many of them are visiting hospitals or general practices up to three days a week, checking progress and data, and providing administrative support (writing reports, answering queries, arranging supplies, etc) for the remainder. Some CRAs work only on one trial in one area of medicine or one geographical region. Others co-ordinate numerous different trials in many therapeutic areas in different countries, even in different languages.

What problems do CRAs face?

The major problem faced by CRAs is that their success depends on the hard work of someone else — namely the investigator — who has a completely different set of priorities. The second problem — shared by the CRA and investigator — is that of the disappearing patient population. The number of patients suitable for a trial during the protocol-writing stage is always reduced by a factor of ten once the supplies are delivered! This has been called Lasagna's Law after a pessimistic, or perhaps experienced, American investigator.

Other problems CRAs experience relate to the different approaches to medicine, in both diagnosis and treatment, in different parts of the world. Measurement techniques and even health care systems vary enormously. If they work for a Japanese or American company who send a fixed protocol over to Europe for a trial with British or French doctors, the CRA may have difficulty persuading investigators to participate in the trial. Similar issues are encountered with CRFs designed in a different culture or country.

CRAs who work with drugs in early phases of development may experience problems or delays in getting permission to conduct the trial, either from ethics committees or national regulatory authorities. It is usually easier when several hundred patients have been successfully treated without mishap. Also, in the early years, the long-term stability of the drug may not yet be established, so CRAs may have problems with deteriorating drug supplies and short shelf-lives.

Like other travelling people, the CRA is vulnerable to motorway jams, air traffic control delays and the other irritations which are the daily lot of executives on the move. Since their appointments are often squeezed in between theatre lists and ward rounds and therefore fairly inflexible, many CRAs experience a high degree of stress.

Who supports the CRA?

Probably the most important source of support for the CRA is their secretary, or personal assistant. You can imagine that being out of the office up to three days a week, they need to be confident that someone competent can handle queries and their administration in their absence and arrange their itinerary thoughtfully. A clinical trials secretary can become familiar with all the investigators, protocols and emergency procedures, and assist with supplies preparation and co-ordination. There should also be opportunities to organize joint investigator meetings and conferences. Many clinical trial secretaries have prior experience in the health service and have studied for the AMSPAR Diploma for Medical Secretaries or equivalent.

Other technical support for the CRA is provided by medical advisers, pharmacists, information scientists, data management staff and statisticians. Drug development is a team exercise and project management skills are vital for a successful programme.

What is a Contract Research Organization?

A **Contract Research Organization** (CRO) is an independent company which undertakes (clinical) research projects on behalf of drug companies. They vary in size and expertise from the small data management or training companies run by a handful of people, to international organizations offering a complete drug development service to the highest standards. The rise in popularity of CROs has followed a harsher economic climate for the pharmaceutical industry with many companies needing to reduce the number of permanent staff, at a time of increased workload per trial. Companies principally employ CROs to monitor, analyse and report trials when they have internal staff shortages or need to conduct trials in a country where they have no staff or experience. Most CROs operate to their own SOPs but interact very closely with the sponsor's medical management. Regulatory authorities (and GCP) accept that sponsors may choose to delegate any or all of the clinical trial process to CROs, but emphasize that the sponsor should ensure that the CRO has adequate facilities and competence.

A CRA working for a CRO will have a very varied life — often working in different therapeutic areas, for several sponsors. Sponsors understandably assume that they will be well-trained and experienced and the trials will all run on schedule. It is therefore a tough environment in which to begin a CRA career.

Why monitor trials?

Thirty years ago the pharmaceutical industry arranged their clinical trials rather informally. Supplies of new drugs were given to experienced doctors who tried them on a series of patients and pronounced on their usefulness. The trials were small and informal, documentation was minimal and the end product was often a paper published in a medical journal.

Now it is different. With increasing requirements for more and more information on new drugs before they are given a licence, drug development has become a much longer and more expensive process. Also the paperwork involved in clinical trials is complex and time-consuming. Generally speaking, the tasks you are reminded about and encouraged in, get done more quickly than those no-one mentions. Doctors are no exception to this. Also, they are used to making independent, sophisticated decisions about diagnosis and treatment without reference to any text-book, so it is not always easy for them to follow a protocol devoutly.

In both these areas, the CRA can benefit the progress of the trial positively. A trial in which a skilled CRA is involved will invariably progress more quickly and with higher quality data than one in which the protocol and trial supplies are posted to a doctor without any follow-up.

How do trials get started?

Once the protocol and CRFs have been designed and the investigators selected, there is a good deal of preparatory work before the trial can start.

First, the protocol must be submitted to the ethics committee for approval. In some cases a central ethics committee (for example the Royal College of General Practitioners Ethics Committee) can be approached directly by the CRA. Local committees must be approached only by the investigator. The chairman or secretary will confirm how many copies of the protocol are needed and the date of the meeting. If the drug is not licensed, the trial and investigator involvement must also be approved by the regulatory authority, eg the MCA. Details of this process can be found in Chapter 2.

The drugs themselves will need to be ordered, packaged and labelled according to national and local regulations. Some trials require the provision of medical equipment and, often, it is the CRA who will organize the ordering, delivery, calibration and maintenance. All the papers which a doctor must sign and keep for reference must be made ready for the 'start up' or initiation meeting. At this meeting the CRA meets the principal investigator to confirm all the final arrangements about the trial agreement (between sponsor and investigator) including protocol, finance, indemnity or insurance. The CVs of investigators will be collected and all the trial supplies (drugs, documentation, CRFs and equipment) delivered and explained (details of trial supplies are discussed in Chapter 7). The CRA will also meet the pharmacist and any other hospital or clinic staff who will be involved. The purpose is to ensure that everyone understands what is required and their respective responsibilities. It is another opportunity for the CRA to answer any questions about the drug or the trial protocol, clarify the trial schedule and establish good communication links with the centre.

Once all the appropriate permissions have been obtained and necessary supplies arranged, the clinical trial can then be started. It is not unusual for the preparation to take three to six months, or even longer with international studies.

How are investigators monitored?

CRAs monitor their trials primarily by supporting the investigator. The first step is to consult the doctors when designing the protocol and CRFs so that these are suitable for the type of patient and disease. If the requested tests and examinations are similar to normal medical practice the research is less likely to go wrong. The CRA's next role is to supply everything the doctor and his staff need to conduct the trial and explain it all: how to fill in the forms, where to send the laboratory samples, when to do each test, etc. If the nurse or junior doctor will actually be doing the work, then the CRA must meet them and provide all possible assistance. The CRA must ensure the investigator knows his legal and ethical responsibilities and agree with every aspect of the clinical trial before it starts.

Once the trial is underway, the CRA will be in touch regularly by telephone and letter and will visit the investigator, usually every four to six weeks, to discuss progress. At these meetings any problems will be reviewed, solutions proposed and the investigator encouraged to give the trial priority. The CRA must check that patients are being enrolled into the trial correctly: for example, that patients of the correct age and disease severity are being recruited, and that no-one with contraindicated (or disallowed) concomitant medication has been entered into the trial by mistake. They must also check for adverse events or inadequate clinical effect, abnormal laboratory test results or any other problems. The trial supplies should be checked to see they are being stored and dispensed properly.

These meetings (and telephone contacts) must be carefully reported and archived by the CRA as part of their monitoring role.

What is data monitoring?

An increasing part of the CRA's job is the checking of completed CRFs. When visiting the investigator, the CRA may spend anything from 30 minutes to several hours reading through the CRFs looking for omissions, inconsistencies or illegible doctors' handwriting(!). This is sometimes called data validation. Before any CRF is collected, all queries should have been corrected by the investigator. The CRA then usually brings the CRF back to the office, checks it again to make sure every page is complete and properly identified, and then passes it to the data-entry staff who enter all the information onto a computer database. Very often, at this stage, further queries are found and relayed back to the CRA, who must return to the investigator and request clarification.

This exacting part of the trial is time-consuming and sometimes very tedious. However, at the end of the trial the only product (apart from patients who have been helped) is a small mountain of coloured paper — or CRFs. You cannot have a high quality study without high quality data.

What is source data verification?

Source data verification (SDV) is the process of checking the trial records or CRFs against the patient's hospital records or GP notes and any other original test results, to prove that the CRF is correct. CRAs must obtain permission to get access to these records. During monitoring visits the CRA then cross checks, with the investigator, certain key information about the patient and their treatment.

What is trial termination?

At the end of a trial, all the CRFs and supplies are collected and the CRA ensures all the necessary payments have been made. The investigator is asked to sign a statement confirming that all the trial patients gave informed consent and that their trial records will be filed securely.

The report or publication will be discussed in principle at this final (trial closure or close-down) meeting. This meeting may mark the end of a three- or four-year collaboration between the CRA and investigator and ideally should be conducted in such a way that both parties will seek an early opportunity to work together again.

A trial may also be 'terminated' prematurely in the case of inadequate patient recruitment (perhaps just at that centre) or if new information causes concerns about the safety or efficacy of the trial drug.

What happens when something goes wrong?

Testing new medicines carries a number of risks: perhaps it does not work as well as expected and people do not get better, perhaps their condition deteriorates; perhaps they suffer undesirable side-effects.

Think of any drug and you will find a group of people who do not benefit from it or are allergic to it. Think of any drug and you can also think of its side-effects. What is acceptable to a patient will depend both on the seriousness of their disease and also on their individual susceptibility to that side-effect.

One problem in developing drugs is discovering whether an undesirable symptom or event experienced by the patient in a drug trial is truly related to the test drug or not. As a result, instead of side-effects, people now tend to refer to adverse events which can include anything that happens to the patient from the beginning to the end of the trial without making any judgement about what caused it. A good understanding of normal physiology, the condition being treated and the drug administered will often enable decisions to be made later about whether or not the drug was responsible.

The investigator is responsible for warning his patients about possible, known, undesirable effects of the trial drugs, and then checking at every visit or assessment for any adverse events. Any adverse events which do occur during a trial must be recorded carefully and reported to the pharmaceutical company.

How are adverse events reported?

Every CRF will have an adverse events section which will guide the investigator to examine the patient or enquire whether they have had any problems since their last visit. The doctor then records the nature of any undesired symptoms, their duration, severity and seriousness. Often the doctor asks about symptoms right at the beginning of the trial to try to establish which symptoms or problems are present before the drug is given. This provides a 'background' for comparison if additional problems occur during the trial. It should be noted, that many people complain of significant adverse events whilst receiving a placebo.

If the doctor has any concerns for the patient, the trial drug treatment should be stopped, and the patient's symptoms monitored carefully.

The CRA or medical adviser should be contacted if the doctor believes an adverse event is serious. Adverse events classified as serious include life-threatening events and those resulting in or prolonging hospitalization and death. Depending on the stage of drug development, the sponsor will then report the adverse event on special forms provided by the drug regulatory authority. Other investigators and their ethics committees may also have to be informed.

Sometimes serious adverse events or a death will result in a clinical trial being suspended or cancelled. It may be that the trial will continue but extra precautions or safety tests will be incorporated. The problems of anticipating and interpreting life-threatening adverse events are highlighted by the fact that for most modern drugs the incidence will be less than one in 20 000 patients and may not be discovered until after the drug has been marketed.

The investigator must have an emergency telephone number where he can contact a medically-qualified drug company employee and discuss any adverse event and subsequent patient care. The investigator must also have access to the code list in a 'blind' trial so that, in an emergency, he/she can quickly establish which drug the patient is taking.

Some drugs are very dangerous when taken in overdose so it is important that they are stored securely and dispensed carefully. Again, if a patient exceeds the dose of a trial drug, the investigator needs immediate access to advice and information, which should be available from the drug company.

What about patient safety?

Patients receiving an unlicensed drug in a clinical trial are, naturally, monitored much more closely than when marketed drugs are presecribed. However, there have been several tragic episodes in the course of recent drug development wherein patients have suffered excessively whilst receiving new drugs on trial. The media are usually quick to expose any supposed error of judgement on the part of the manufacturer or researcher. These experiences have resulted in individual doctors and some health authorities refusing to participate in clinical trials with new drugs unless the manufacturer provides comprehensive indemnity/insurance cover. This confirms that, should a patient attempt to sue the doctor, the pharmaceutical company will accept responsibility, providing there was no medical negligence and the protocol was followed properly.

Analysis and Reports

10

How are trial results analysed?

Once all the patients have been studied and the CRFs completed, the trial enters analysis, ie the figures are examined and interpreted.

It is hoped that analysis will enable conclusions to be drawn, and the trial to have a definite outcome. Examples would be: drug A works better than drug B, or drug A and drug B are equally effective but drug B causes more side-effects. Sometimes a negative conclusion will be drawn, eg drug A is no better than a placebo or showed no benefit to the patients treated.

The trial findings are usually entered from the CRF directly into a computer — this is called data entry — and tables are made of all the data.

The trial patients are then described, eg 27 males and 33 females with an average age of 45 in Group 1, and 24 males and 36 females with an average age of 41 in Group 2. Similarly, duration and severity of disease and other relevant factors will be examined and described. Before the effects of the drugs on the groups of patients can be compared you must establish that each group was comparable at the beginning of the trial.

Once the patient's background (or demography) is described you would look at the results for the various assessments made at each visit. Almost immediately the analysis can run into problems, for whilst every patient is likely to have age and sex recorded, not everyone will have attended for every single assessment. When the data are being examined you have to decide what to do about the gaps — a patient could have missed a visit because he was ill, or missed the bus or felt cured. Similarly, patients drop out of trials for a variety of reasons: adverse events, because they felt their condition was worse on the test drug or no better, because they were 'cured' or perhaps because they did not like the measurement techniques/the doctor's manner/the taste, etc. Sometimes you know why results are missing, more often you do not, and therefore you cannot assume the results that day would be better, worse or the same as at the previous visit. Very often the analysis of why and how many patients withdrew from the trial can be the most important outcome of a trial of a new drug.

Essentially, there are three basic ways of looking at the results:

1 compare the proportion of patients showing a particular response, eg 15/30 were cured in Group 1 at week 8 and 23/30 in Group 2

2 compare the average results for each group

3 look at the difference between the first and last result for each patient, and compare these for each group.

What are statistics?

Statistics are the collection and organization of numerical facts or data. The word derives from the Greek 'statis', meaning the state, as statistics were originally figures collated for the state, eg a population census. Ideally, they can help describe numerically the findings of a clinical trial.

A well-known statistic is the mean or average; another common way of describing the mid-point of a series of figures is the median which is literally the middle number if they were arranged in ascending order. The mode is the most frequently occurring number in a series. Another useful descriptive statistic is the range.

For example, supposing you wished to describe the ages of a small trial in seven children; it would be usual to talk about an average and range:

Ages:　　4　7　7　8　9　10　11 years
　　　　　Mean = 56 ÷ 7 = 8
　　　　　Median = 8
　　　　　Mode = 7
Range = 4–11

Is the result significant?

When an experiment is conducted and a result obtained it is important to be able to interpret the relevance. In drug development you have to ask 'is it of any clinical significance?'. This decision is up to the clinician and has very little to do with statistics. However, any scientist also wishes to know 'could the result have happened by chance?'. You would like to think that the clinical trial is conducted on a representative sample of the patient population, but it is necessarily a highly selected sample. Perhaps the same trial done with a different sample would produce a different result. It is usual to apply significance tests to data to establish the probability (p) of the result being a chance finding. It is beyond the scope of this book to describe the different tests habitually employed for clinical trials data. However, when reading about clinical trials you will see the expression 'a statistically significant result' and this usually refers to a p value of less than 5% — which means less than a 5% likelihood of the result arising by chance.

How are reports prepared?

Clinical trial reports may be statistical or clinical — statistical reports describe the analysis and the results of any significance tests applied to them. Clinical reports describe the clinical context and relevance of the results and discuss the wider implications, eg in comparison to other treatments, the importance of reported side-effects etc.

These reports are often prepared by statisticians and medical advisers — either as part of the pharmaceutical company or external contractors. Reports are also commonly prepared by CRAs and project leaders in clinical trial departments or regulatory affairs personnel. If the trial has been performed to provide evidence in support of a PL it will be structured in a specific way to suit the regulatory authority. In addition, most companies have their own in-house style. Usually trial reports contain the following elements:

▼ trial investigators and identification
▼ introduction and rationale
▼ methods: patient selection criteria, drugs, measurements (clinical and laboratory), statistical analysis
▼ results: demography, safety, efficacy, withdrawals etc
▼ discussion
▼ conclusions
▼ data tables (appended)
▼ protocol (appended).

The final report should be signed by the author, investigators, statistician and responsible medical adviser for the company.

Although most reports are prepared after trial completion, for some long-term trials a brief annual report may be prepared for the regulatory authorities or ethics committee. The annual report focuses on trial progress and any adverse events. Interim reports may be produced at certain key points in the trial, but this is unusual.

What about publication of trial results?

Most researchers and drug companies are keen to publicize encouraging results with their new drug. Very often junior doctors need a few respectable published papers to achieve promotion. As a result, clinical trials with positive results are frequently published as papers in medical journals or as verbal presentations at academic medical conferences.

Papers must be written in a specified style to suit the journal of choice. Prestigious journals such as *The Lancet* and the *British Medical Journal* have expert editors who review papers for scientific interest and originality and may take many months to publish a paper. Some clinical trials are of more commercial than scientific merit and these may only find their way into print promptly if a 'paying' journal is approached. These have fewer editorial limitations and survive by printing drug trial reports.

Drug companies often favour holding a small symposium to discuss and publicize the development of a new drug. Medical opinion leaders are usually invited to hear a series of papers presented by investigators. These are later published as symposium 'proceedings'. Not infrequently, these symposia are arranged by the medical department staff once the PLA is submitted for the new drug. CRAs and medical secretaries may find themselves organizing travel and venues as well as typing and proof-reading abstracts and papers for publication and preparing slides. Although time-consuming, these events may be the culmination of many years of hard work in clinical trials with the new drug and can be a satisfying and sociable way to finalize the programme.

11

Standard Operating Procedures (SOPs), Audits and Archives

What are standard operating procedures?

One of the more recent abbreviations to hit the clinical trials scene is SOP (standard operating procedure), which is, literally, a step-by-step guide to the standard way things are done in a company or clinical trials department. People have been writing down common procedures and instructions since script was invented, but SOPs have only relatively recently been introduced by the drug regulatory authorities and industry for laboratory, manufacturing and research practices. The possession of SOPs for all clinical trial activities is a vital requirement if you are to comply with GCP. As mentioned in Chapter 3, most companies aspire to achieve GCP standards so that authorities all over the world will accept and respect the quality of their drug research work.

You would normally have SOPs for such key activities as protocol-writing, monitoring, adverse event reporting, drug accountability, data management, study reporting and archiving. Often companies have SOPs for many other activities as well.

Who needs SOPs?

If SOPs are written in a fluent and readable way, they can be a very helpful addition to a department's training material. If new members of staff join the department, let them read the SOPs and they will have an immediate idea not only of what is done, but by whom and how. Usually, comprehensive SOPs grow into mighty tomes which may be too daunting to read all at once but which provide an ideal reference if you need to know specific information. This can be a great help for all those times when you only think of the question when there is no-one there to ask, or you have already asked ten things that morning and cannot bring yourself to do it again! Complex SOPs usually have accompanying checklists or aide-mémoires which simplify matters.

Therefore SOPs are useful to new staff, people who cannot keep all the details of a complex job in their head, managers and finally the auditors or quality assurance staff. The latter have the job of reporting whether everyone is following the SOPs or simply 'doing their own thing'.

Why have clinical trial audit?

You will be accustomed to the accounts of a company being audited by an independent group who report on financial irregularities and generally on the way the books are kept. Audit of clinical trials has been introduced for the same reason. Just occasionally someone gets over-enthusiastic about the virtues of their drugs and rarely (but it still happens) someone cheats. It could happen that an investigator forgets to make some measurements and invents them later to keep the CRFs complete, or even that a CRA is negligent and does not report adverse events properly.

So it was deemed sensible to have some unbiased observer examining the records of a trial and reporting any deviation from the protocol or company SOPs. This practice is relatively recent in Europe — the GCP guidelines, which include the requirement for independent audit, were only introduced in 1992 and have not yet been fully implemented by all drug companies.

How will you be audited?

Most clinical trial audits are performed routinely at a pre-arranged date and in a predictable way — indeed there should be an SOP for audits! The auditors will arrange to visit the department and will either request a particular set of archives to be made available, or will arrange an audit of an investigator at their clinic. They may wish to check drug accountability records, sample storage, laboratory procedures and/or source data verification. Data managed, the appropriate use of computers and reporting procedures should also be audited.

Whatever the subject, the auditors prepare a comprehensive report which is usually sent to the medical directors and senior managers. No one enjoys being checked up on, but clinical trials audit may improve the safety of drug trials and certainly increases their acceptance by regulatory authorities. Auditors will often have helpful ideas about how to improve standards and procedures.

Occasionally, a company may have anxieties about the quality or validity of an investigator's data. They can request the company quality assurance staff to conduct a thorough site-audit to provide an independent view of standards.

In some countries, the drug regulatory authority has a team of inspectors who conduct audits on investigators and pharmaceutical companies' trial records. They will examine SOPs, cross-check the CRFs and trial reports against patient records and compile an extensive quality assurance report. The FDA has been following this practice, throughout the world, for many years and European countries are now following their example.

Where should all this information be kept?

With the increasing emphasis on carefully documenting all trials activities, it is very important that filing and archiving are done well. The secretary or office manager should be responsible for creating and maintaining scrupulous files for all the medico-legal documents, correspondence, reports and patient data. Some companies keep these originals together in a Trial Master File. Most trial files will have the following subsections:

▼ originals of protocol and CRFs
▼ investigator details
▼ monitoring reports and correspondence
▼ finances
▼ drug accountability records
▼ adverse events
▼ code lists
▼ ethical and legal letters (eg approvals, indemnities, contracts)
▼ trial results and reports.

Completed CRFs, queries and other original patient data such as laboratory reports are usually filed separately, often in fire-resistant containers. Certain documents must be retained for inspection as long as the drug is on the market, in case a regulatory authority raises questions (in the future) and then all the research data might need re-examining. Therefore, on trial completion, the CRFs and important trial documents must be archived carefully.

Appendix:
Glossary of Abbreviations

ABPI	Association of the British Pharmaceutical Industry
ACRPI	Association for Clinical Research in the Pharmaceutical Industry
ADE	Adverse drug event
ADR	Adverse drug reaction
AE	Adverse event
AICRC	Association of Independent Clinical Research Contractors
BMJ	British Medical Journal
BP	British Pharmacopoeia
CPMP	Committee for Proprietary Medicinal Products
CRA	Clinical Research Associate
CRF	Case record form or report
CRO	Contract Research Organization
CSM	Committee on Safety of Medicines
CTC	Clinical Trial Certificate
CTX	Clinical Trial Certificate Exemption
CV	Curriculum vitae
FDA	Food and Drug Administration (USA regulatory authority)
GCP	Good Clinical Practice (sometimes called Good Clinical Research Practice)
GLP	Good Laboratory Practice
GMP	Good Manufacturing Practice
IND	Notice of claimed investigational exemption for a new drug
IRB	Institutional Review Board (ethics committee)
MCA	Medicines Control Agency

PLA	Product Licence Application
PMS	Post-marketing surveillance
SDV	Source data verification
SHO	Senior House Officer
SOP	Standard operating procedure
SR	Senior registrar
TMF	Trial Master File

Abbreviations of common medical qualifications and how to use them can be found in Appendix 4, page 75.

Appendix:
Glossary of Terms

Adverse drug reaction (ADR) — adverse events that are considered to be caused by a trial drug.

Adverse event — any undesirable experience (occurring during a clinical trial), whether or not it is considered to be drug-related (*see also* serious adverse event).

Analogues — drugs which are similar or come from the same family.

Animal models — artificially-created animal preparations which mimic a medical condition, designed to test the effects of new drugs.

Audit (of a trial) — a comparison of source data and associated records with the trial report to determine whether the trial has been accurately reported. In addition, an audit should check whether the trial was carried out in accordance with the protocol and the SOPs.

Bias — an opinion, feeling or influence that strongly favours one aspect (or treatment) when there is a choice (treatment bias may be exhibited by doctors or patients, or both).

Black list (of investigators) — a list of investigators compiled by a company or regulatory authority whose data are not deemed acceptable and who will not be invited to collaborate in clinical trials. The FDA also produce a list of investigators who have been 'blacklisted'.

Blind — a term used to describe a trial in which the patient or the investigator (and sometimes both) do not know what trial medication is being taken by the patient (*see also* single blind and double blind).

Carcinogenicity — potential to cause cancer.

Case record form or case report form (CRF) — a document which reflects the protocol and provides for the recording of all trial data for an individual subject.

Clinical significance — a result from a trial which is of clinical relevance.

Close down — the act of terminating a trial. Sites may be closed down because the trial has been completed or for safety or procedural reasons.

Concomitant medication — drugs (excluding the trial drugs) being taken by a patient during a clinical trial. They may have been prescribed for a different condition.

Contraindicated — treatments which are not permitted (during a clinical trial). Certain drugs are contraindicated for subgroups of patients for reasons of safety.

Contract Research Organization (CRO) — an institution or company (commercial or academic) to which a drug company may transfer some responsibility of the drug development process, eg trial monitoring, data analysis.

Controlled trial — groups of patients are managed in an identical manner with the exception of treatment received, and the responses are compared.

Crossover study — individual patients receive both treatments one after another and their responses are compared.

Data entry — the process of transcribing the contents of a CRF onto a computer database for the purpose of analysis.

Demography — a description of the features of the trial population: their racial and physical characteristics, age patterns, disease history, etc.

Double blind — a trial in which neither the assessor (usually the doctor) nor the patient are aware of which treatment has been allocated.

Double dummy — a procedure for achieving blindness when comparing two unlike drugs wherein, for example, an active injection and placebo tablet are given to one group and the matching placebo injection and active tablet are given to the other group.

Ethics committee — an independent body, including medical and non-medical members who consider clinical trials in the context of safety, integrity and human rights.

Expert report — a report required by the regulatory authorities regarding some aspect of a drug (eg toxicology, chemistry and pharmacy, clinical). The author of such a report must be an expert in that particular field and may be a company employee or an external person.

Good Clinical Practice — a standard by which clinical trials are designed, implemented and reported so that there is public assurance that the data are credible, and that the rights, integrity and confidentiality of subjects are protected.

Group comparison — a trial design in which patients are randomly allocated to either of two or more treatment groups and the responses of each group are compared.

Investigator — a medically-qualified person responsible for the practical performance of a trial and for the welfare of the patient.

Investigator brochure — a booklet of all the relevant information known prior to the onset of a clinical trial including: chemical and pharmaceutical data, toxicological and pharmacological data in animals and the results of earlier clinical trials. There should be adequate data to justify the nature, scale and duration of the clinical study. The brochure should be updated during the course of drug development.

Indication — condition or disease which a drug is intended to treat.

Mean — the arithmetic average which is obtained by dividing the sum of the measurements by the number of measurements.

Median — the middle number when all the measurements are arranged in rank order.

Mode — the most frequently occurring value.

Monitor — a person appointed by the sponsor or CRO who is responsible to the sponsor (or CRO) for the monitoring and reporting on the progress of the trial and for verification of data. The monitor must have the qualifications and the experience to enable a knowledgeable supervision of a clinical trial. Trained technical assistants may help the monitor in the collection of documentation and subsequent processing.

Multicentre trial — a clinical trial conducted according to one protocol, but in several different locations and therefore involving different investigators.

Named patient basis — an unlicensed drug being supplied to a doctor for use in a particular patient. The drug supply cannot be used for any other patient. The patient should be monitored carefully and a brief report supplied to the drug company.

Normal range — the range of values for a specific (usually laboratory) parameter which are considered clinically normal. These will vary slightly depending on the laboratory and are used as a reference against which individual patients' results are compared.

Open — a term used to describe a trial in which both the patient and the assessor are aware of the treatment being allocated.

Patient population — relating to patients: the total number of people suffering from a particular condition or disease.

Pharmacology — the science of the properties of drugs and their effects on the body.

Pharmacokinetics — study of the time course of absorption, distribution, metabolism and excretion of drugs by the body.

Phase I — first trials of a new drug in man, usually conducted in healthy volunteers.

Phase II — early efficacy and safety trials conducted in limited numbers of patients. They include dose-finding studies to establish an appropriate range of doses.

Phase III — major efficacy and safety trials in large numbers of patients. Ideally the circumstances of the trials should be close to normal conditions of use for the new drug.

Phase IV — trials performed after marketing of the drug, in indications for which it is licensed.

Physiology — the scientific study of the functioning of the body and all constituent systems.

Pilot study — a mini-study conducted in advance of the main experiment, usually to assess feasibility.

Placebo — an inert substance, with no pharmacological activity which is made up to look like a medicine. It is ineffective but may help the patient's condition because they have faith in its powers. New drugs are tested against placebos in clinical trials.

Placebo response — a patient's clinical response whilst receiving placebo treatment.

Post-marketing surveillance — large Phase IV studies conducted to evaluate further the safety profile of a new drug, after a PL has been granted.

Power — the likelihood that a trial design will be able to detect a real difference, when it exists.

Preclinical — referring to (research) activities prior to research in patients.

Probability (p) — the likelihood (eg of 5% or less) that an observed difference could have arisen by chance.

Protocol — a document which states the rationale, objectives, design and methodology of the trial, with the conditions under which it is to be performed and managed.

Randomize — relating to allocation of patients to a treatment: the process which ensures that each patient is allocated to different treatments in an unpredictable manner.

Regulatory authority — a government body, consisting of scientific experts and administrators who control the use of medicines and research on new drugs.

Run-in — a period at the beginning of a clinical trial during which no active trial drug is provided, often used to reduce (effects of) previous treatments, or to establish baseline severity of illness/eligibility for the trial.

Sample — a sub-group or selection of patients which should be representative of the patient population.

Scale-up — expansion of the manufacturing process of a new drug from research-sized batches to commercial production.

Serious adverse event — an adverse experience that is fatal, life-threatening, disabling or which results in patient hospitalization or prolongation of hospitalization. In addition, congenital anomaly and occurrence of malignancy are always considered serious adverse events.

Significance tests — tests applied to a set of data which seek to establish whether the results could have occurred by chance and therefore their 'significance'.

Single blind — a term used to describe a trial in which either the assessor (usually the doctor) or the patient, but not both, are aware of which treatment has been allocated.

Statistical significance — statistical test result in which p is less than or equal to 0.05 (ie a 5% probability of the result occurring by chance).

Teratology — the study of developmental abnormalities and their cause.

Toxicology — the study of poisons, eg drugs, and their effects on plants and animals.

Toxicity — the degree to which a substance is poisonous.

Trial Master File — a file or archive containing all the key documents as defined by GCP guidelines.

Washout — a treatment-free period either at the outset of a clinical trial or between two treatments of a cross-over trial. The purpose is to remove the effects of the previous treatment or avoid drug interactions.

Appendix: Further Reading/ Resource Material

Guidelines

Clinical Trials — Compensation for Medicine-induced Injury. ABPI (January 1991).

Code of Practice for the Clinical Assessment of Licensed Medicinal Products in General Practice. ABPI (November 1992).

Declaration of Helsinki. See Appendix 7, page 81.

Fraud and Malpractice in the Context of Clinical Research. ABPI (May 1992).

Good Clinical Practice for Trials on Medicinal Products in the European Community. Document III/3976/88-EN, Final 11.07.1990. *See* Appendix 8, page 85.

Guidelines for Medical Experiments in Non-patient Human Volunteers. ABPI (May 1989).

Guidelines on Good Clinical Research Practice. ABPI (September 1992).

Guidelines on the Practice of Ethics Committees in Medical Research. Royal College of Physicians of London (1990).

Research Involving Patients. Royal College of Physicians of London (1990).

Books

British National Formulary (BNF). Published jointly by the British Medical Association and the Royal Pharmaceutical Society. (A manual listing details of all marketed drugs available in the UK, arranged according to therapeutic area, published regularly.)

Concise Medical Dictionary. Oxford University Press, Oxford.

Data Sheet Compendium. ABPI (annually). (A comprehensive list, per company, of prescribing information on drugs marketed in the UK.)

Lloyd J and Raven A (1994) *ACRPI Handbook of Clinical Drug Research*, 2nd Ed. Churchill Livingstone, Edinburgh. (A comprehensive textbook on clinical drug development, written primarily for CRAs.) In press.

Riddle J (1985) *Anatomy and Physiology Applied to Nursing*. Churchill Livingstone, Edinburgh. (A well-structured simple introduction to the subject, suitable for programmed learning.)

Sneader W (1986) *Drug Development: from laboratory to clinic*. Wiley, Chichester. (A concise paperback describing the breadth of the drug development process.)

The Medical Directory, Longmans, London. (A two volume directory of UK doctors, published annually.)

Associations

Association for Clinical Research in the Pharmaceutical Industry
This is an association primarily for CRAs. It has a regular journal, publishes educational material and provides

information on CRA careers. Also there are conferences and workshops organized on a regular basis. Further details available from ACRPI, PO Box 1208, Maidenhead, Berks SL6 2YH. Tel: 0628 29617

Association of Clinical Data Management (ACDM)
PO Box 1208, Maidenhead, Berks SL6 2YH. Tel: 0628 789450

Association of the British Pharmaceutical Industry (ABPI)
12 Whitehall, London, SW1A 2DY. Tel: 071 930 3477

Association of Independent Clinical Research Contractors (AICRC)
Department of Pharmacology and Therapeutics, University of Wales College of Medicine, Heath Park, Cardiff CF4 4XN. Tel: 0222 747747 Ext 2353

Association of Information Officers in the Pharmaceutical Industry (AIOPI)
Glaxo Pharmaceuticals UK Ltd, Building 10, Stockley Park West, Uxbridge, Middx UB11 1BT. Tel: 081 990 9000

Association of Medical Secretaries, Practice Administrators and Receptionists (AMSPAR)
Tavistock House North, Tavistock Square, London WC1H 9LN. Tel: 071 387 6005. This is a professional association for a range of administrative staff working in the field; several courses and qualifications are available.

The British Institute of Regulatory Affairs (BIRA)
34 Dover Street, London W1X 3RA. Tel: 071 499 2797

Society of Pharmaceutical Medicine
1 Wimpole Street, London W1M 8AE. Tel: 071 491 8610

Statisticians in the Pharmaceutical Industry (PSI)
Mrs Carol McKellar, PO Box 37, Ely, Cambs CB6 3XY. Tel: 0353 648740

Appendix:
Use of Medical
Qualifications (UK)

The guidelines for adding letters after a name in formal medical correspondence are as follows.

1 Honours and decorations come before university degrees and diplomas:
   Sir Adam Haig, KBE, FRCS, *or*
   Adam Haig Esq., OBE, FRCS

2 Medical degrees are placed before surgical:
   Adam Haig, Esq., MD, FRCS

3 Surgical degrees take precedence over degrees in obstetrics and gynaecology:
   Adam Haig, Esq., FRCS, FRCOG

   A surgeon's MD should *always* be featured in his degrees

4 When postgraduate degrees are held, qualifying degrees may be omitted, eg Mr J Dunn, FRCS (omitting his qualifying degree of MB, ChB)

   Once MD qualification awarded, qualifying degrees are omitted, eg J Dunn, MD, FRCS and *not* J Dunn, MB, ChB, MD, FRCOG

5 University degrees take precedence over the qualifications of the Royal Colleges, which precede diplomas, eg Mr J Dunn, MB, ChB, MSc, FRCS, DMR

Although 'Esquire' has more or less been dropped in the commercial world, it is recommended as a useful term to be used when writing to the medical profession.

Appendix: Commonly Used Qualifications (UK)

BAO	Bachelor of the Art of Obstetrics
BCh/BChir/BS/ChB	Bachelor of Surgery
BM	Bachelor of Medicine
BSc	Bachelor of Science
CM, ChM	Master of Surgery
DCh	Doctor of Surgery
Dip.Pharm.Med	Diploma in Pharmaceutical Medicine
DM	Doctor of Medicine
DObst RCOG	Diploma in Obstetrics of the Royal College of Obstetricians and Gynaecologists
DPhysMed	Diploma in Physical Medicine
FRCGP	Fellow of Royal College of General Practitioners
FRCOG	Fellow of Royal College of Obstetricians and Gynaecologists
FRCP	Fellow of Royal College of Physicians of London
FRCPE*	Fellow of Royal College of Physicians of Edinburgh
FRCPGlasg.	Fellow of Royal College of Physicians and Surgeons of Glasgow
FRCPath	Fellow of Royal College of Pathologists
FRCPsych	Fellow of Royal College of Psychiatrists
FRCS	Fellow of Royal College of Surgeons
FRCSE*	Fellow of Royal College of Surgeons of Edinburgh
FRS	Fellow of Royal Society
LMS	Licentiate in Medicine and Surgery

LMSSA	Licentiate in Medicine and Surgery, Society of Apothecaries
LRCP	Licentiate of Royal College of Physicians
MAO	Master of the Art of Obstetrics
MB	Bachelor of Medicine
MC/MCh/MChir	Master of Surgery
MCh/Orth	Master of Orthopaedic Surgery
MD	Doctor of Medicine
MRCGP	Member of Royal College of General Practitioners
MRCOG	Member of Royal College of Obstetricians and Gynaecologists
MRCP Ed	Member of Royal College of Physicians and Surgeons of Edinburgh
MRCP Glasg.	Member of Royal College of Physicians and Surgeons of Glasgow
MRCP (UK)	Member of Royal College of Physicians
MRCPath	Member of Royal College of Pathologists
MRCPsych	Member of Royal College of Psychiatrists
MRCS	Member of Royal College of Surgeons
MS	Master of Surgery

*This may be written as FRCP(Ed.), FRCP.Ed, FRCP(Edin.) or FRCPE. It is correct to add the appropriate college after the MRCP, FRCP or FRCS of the Scottish Royal Colleges.

Appendix: Questions for Group Discussion

Chapters 1–3

▼ What are the different sources of new drugs?
▼ Why are trials done in healthy volunteers?
▼ What is the role of a regulatory authority?
▼ What do ethics committees do?
▼ Describe informed consent and how it should be obtained?
▼ Why have drug companies adopted GCP?

Chapters 4–7

▼ How is an investigator selected?
▼ Why do doctors become investigators?
▼ What is the power of a clinical trial?
▼ Why are placebos used in drug trials?
▼ What is a double dummy design?
▼ What is a pilot study and why would one be conducted?
▼ Who should be consulted when CRFs are designed?
▼ What are the key elements of a CRF?
▼ What are the advantages of a central pathology laboratory for a multicentre trial?
▼ What is an investigator brochure?

Chapters 8 – 11

▼ What personal attributes does a good CRA need?
▼ What are a CRA's principle responsibilities?
▼ What should trial monitoring achieve?
▼ What happens at an initiation meeting?
▼ Why is SDV performed?
▼ What are significance tests?
▼ Why are SOPs used for clinical trials?
▼ Why are clinical trials audited?

Appendix: World Medical Association Declaration of Helsinki: recommendations guiding physicians in biomedical research involving human subjects

7

Adopted by the 18th World Medical Assembly Helsinki, Finland, June 1964; and amended by the 29th World Medical Assembly Tokyo, Japan, October 1975; 35th World Medical Assembly Venice, Italy, October 1983 and the 41st World Medical Assembly Hong Kong, September 1989.

Introduction

It is the mission of the physician to safeguard the health of the people. His or her knowledge and conscience are dedicated to the fulfilment of this mission.

The Declaration of Geneva of the World Medical Association binds the physician with the words, 'The health of my patient will be my first consideration,' and the International Code of Medical Ethics declares that, 'A physician shall act only in the patient's interest when providing medical care which might have the effect of weakening the physical and mental condition of the patient.'

The purpose of biomedical research involving human subjects must be to improve diagnostic, therapeutic and prophylactic procedures and the understanding of the aetiology and pathogenesis of disease.

In current medical practice most diagnostic, therapeutic or prophylactic procedures involve hazards. This applies especially to biomedical research.

Medical progress is based on research which ultimately must rest in part on experimentation involving human subjects.

In the field of biomedical research a fundamental distinction must be recognized between medical research in which the aim is essentially diagnostic or therapeutic for a patient, and medical research, the essential object of which is purely scientific and without implying direct diagnostic or therapeutic value to the person subjected to the research.

Special caution must be exercised in the conduct of research which may affect the environment, and the welfare of animals used for research must be respected.

Because it is essential that the results of laboratory experiments be applied to human beings to further scientific knowledge and to help suffering humanity, the World Medical Association has prepared the following recommendations as a guide to every physician in biomedical research involving human subjects. They should be kept under review in the future. It must be stressed that the standards as drafted are only a guide to physicians all over the world. Physicians are not relieved from criminal, civil and ethical responsibilities under the laws of their own countries.

I. Basic Principles

1. Biomedical research involving human subjects must conform to generally accepted scientific principles and should be based on adequately performed laboratory and animal experimentation and on a thorough knowledge of the scientific literature.
2. The design and performance of each experimental procedure involving human subjects should be clearly formulated in an experimental protocol which should be transmitted for consideration, comment and guidance to a specially appointed committee independent of the investigator and the sponsor provided that this independent committee is in conformity with the laws and regulations of the country in which the research experiment is performed.
3. Biomedical research involving human subjects should be conducted only by scientifically qualified persons and under the supervision of a clinically competent medical person. The responsibility for the human subject must always rest with a medically qualified person and never rest on the subject of the research, even though the subject has given his or her consent.
4. Biomedical research involving human subjects cannot legitimately be carried out unless the importance of the objective is in proportion to the inherent risk to the subject.
5. Every biomedical research project involving human subjects should be preceded by careful assessment of predictable risks in comparison with foreseeable benefits to the subject or to others. Concern for the interests of the subject must always prevail over the interests of science and society.

6. The right of the research subject to safeguard his or her integrity must always be respected. Every precaution should be taken to respect the privacy of the subject and to minimize the impact of the study on the subject's physical and mental integrity and on the personality of the subject.

7. Physicians should abstain from engaging in research projects involving human subjects unless they are satisfied that the hazards involved are believed to be predictable. Physicians should cease any investigation if the hazards are found to outweigh the potential benefits.

8. In publication of the results of his or her research, the physician is obliged to preserve the accuracy of the results. Reports of experimentation not in accordance with the principles laid down in this Declaration should not be accepted for publication.

9. In any research on human beings, each potential subject must be adequately informed of the aims, methods, anticipated benefits and potential hazards of the study and the discomfort it may entail. He or she should be informed that he or she is at liberty to abstain from participation in the study and that he or she is free to withdraw his or her consent to participation at any time. The physician should then obtain the subject's freely-given informed consent, preferably in writing.

10. When obtaining informed consent for the research project the physician should be particularly cautious if the subject is in a dependent relationship to him or her or may consent under duress. In that case the informed consent should be obtained by a physician who is not engaged in the investigation and who is completely independent of this official relationship.

11. In case of legal incompetence, informed consent should be obtained from the legal guardian in accordance with national legislation. Where physical or mental incapacity makes it impossible to obtain informed consent, or when the subject is a minor, permission from the responsible relative replaces that of the subject in accordance with national legislation.

    Whenever the minor child is in fact able to give a consent, the minor's consent must be obtained in addition to the consent of the minor's legal guardian.

12. The research protocol should always contain a statement of the ethical considerations involved and should indicate that the principles enunciated in the present Declaration are complied with.

II. Medical Research Combined with Professional Care (Clinical research)

1. In the treatment of the sick person, the physician must be free to use a new diagnostic and therapeutic measure, if in his or her judgement it offers hope of saving life, re-establishing health or alleviating suffering.
2. The potential benefits, hazards and discomfort of a new method should be weighed against the advantages of the best current diagnostic and therapeutic methods.
3. In any medical study, every patient — including those of a control group, if any — should be assured of the best proven diagnostic and therapeutic method.
4. The refusal of the patient to participate in a study must never interfere with the physician–patient relationship.
5. If the physician considers it essential not to obtain informed consent, the specific reasons for this proposal should be stated in the experimental protocol for transmission to the independent committee (I,2).
6. The physician can combine medical research with professional care, the objective being the acquisition of new medical knowledge, only to the extent that medical research is justified by its potential diagnostic or therapeutic value for the patient.

III. Non-therapeutic Biomedical Research Involving Human Subjects (Non-clinical biomedical research)

1. In the purely scientific application of medical research carried out on a human being, it is the duty of the physician to remain the protector of the life and health of that person on whom biomedical research is being carried out.
2. The subjects should be volunteers — either healthy persons or patients for whom the experimental design is not related to the patient's illness.
3. The investigator or the investigating team should discontinue the research if in his/her or their judgement it may, if continued, be harmful to the individual.
4. In research on man, the interest of science and society should never take precedence over considerations related to the wellbeing of the subject.

Appendix:
EC Note for Guidance:
Good Clinical Practice for Trials
on Medicinal Products in the
European Community

8

Chapter 1: Protection of Trial Subjects and Consultation of Ethics Committees

PROTECTION OF TRIAL SUBJECTS

1.1 The current revision of the Declaration of Helsinki is the accepted basis for clinical trial ethics, which must be fully known and followed by all engaged in research on human beings.

1.2 The personal integrity and welfare of the trial subjects is the ultimate responsibility of the investigator in relation to the trial; but independent assurance that subjects are protected is provided by an Ethics Committee and freely obtained informed consent.

ETHICS COMMITTEES

1.3 The sponsor and/or investigator must request the opinion of relevant Ethics Committee(s) regarding suitability of clinical trial protocols (including annexes) and of the methods and material to be used in obtaining and documenting informed consent of the subjects.

1.4 The Ethics Committee must be informed of all subsequent protocol amendments and of serious or unexpected AEs occurring during the trial, likely to affect the safety of the subjects or the conduct of the trial, and should be asked for its opinion if a re-evaluation of the ethical aspects of the trial appears to be called for.

1.5 Subjects must not be entered into the trial until the relevant Ethics Committee(s) has issued its favourable opinion on the procedures and documentation. Sponsor/investigator should consider recommendations made by the Ethics Committee.

1.6 In submitting clinical trial proposals to an Ethics Committee, they should be asked to consider the following:

   a) the suitability of the investigator for the proposed trial in relation to his/her qualifications, experience, supporting staff, and available facilities, on basis of the information available to the Committee.

b) the suitability of the protocol in relation to the objectives of the study, its scientific efficiency ie the potential for reaching sound conclusions with the smallest possible exposure of subjects, and the justification of predictable risks and inconveniences weighed against the anticipated benefits for the subjects and/or others.

c) the adequacy and completeness of the written information to be given to the subjects, their relatives, guardians and, if necessary, legal representatives.

d) the means by which initial recruitment is to be conducted and by which full information is to be given, and by which consent is to be obtained. All written information for the subject and/or legal representative must be submitted in its final form.

e) provision for compensation/treatment in the case of injury or death of a subject if attributable to a clinical trial, and any insurance or indemnity to cover the liability of the investigator and sponsor.

f) the extent to which investigators and subjects may be rewarded/compensated for participation.

1.7 The Ethics Committee should give its opinion and advice in writing within a reasonable time limit, clearly identifying the trial, the documents studied and date of review.

INFORMED CONSENT

1.8 The principles of informed consent in the current revision of the Helsinki Declaration should be implemented in each clinical trial.

1.9 Information should be given in both oral and written form whenever possible. No subject should be obliged to participate in the trial. Subjects, their relatives, guardians or, if necessary, legal representatives must be given ample opportunity to enquire about details of the trial. The information must make clear that refusal to participate or withdrawal from the trial at any stage is without any disadvantages for the subject's subsequent care. Subjects must be allowed sufficient time to decide whether or not they wish to participate.

1.10 The subject must be made aware and consent that personal information may be scrutinized during audit by competent authorities and properly authorized persons, but that personal information will be treated as strictly confidential and not be publicly available.

1.11　The subject must have access to information about the procedures for compensation and treatment should he/she be injured/disabled by participating in the trial.

1.12　If a subject consents to participate after a full and comprehensive explanation of the study (including its aims, expected benefits for the subjects and/or others, reference treatments/placebo, risks and inconveniences — eg invasive procedures — and, where appropriate, an explanation of alternative, recognized standard medical therapy), this consent should be appropriately recorded. Consent must be documented either by the subject's dated signature or by the signature of an independent witness who records the subject's assent. In either case the signature confirms that the consent is based on information which has been understood, and that the subject has freely chosen to participate without prejudice to legal and ethical rights while allowing the possibility of withdrawal from the study without having to give any reason unless AEs have occurred.

1.13　If the subject is incapable of giving personal consent (eg unconsciousness or severe mental illness or disability), the inclusion of such patients may be acceptable if the Ethics Committee is, in principle, in agreement and if the investigator is of the opinion that participation will promote the welfare and interest of the subject. The agreement of a legally valid representative that participation will promote the welfare and interest of the subject should also be recorded by a dated signature. If neither signed informed consent nor witnessed signed verbal consent are possible, this fact must be documented with reasons by the investigator.

1.14　Consent must always be given by the signature of the subject in a non-therapeutic study, ie when there is no direct clinical benefit to the subject.

1.15　Any information becoming available during the trial which may be of relevance for the trial subjects must be made known to them by the investigator.

Chapter 2:　Responsibilities

Note: Responsibilities related to data handling, archiving, statistics and assurance of quality are included in subsequent chapters.

SPONSOR

2.1　The sponsor must establish detailed Standard Operating Procedures (SOP) to comply with Good Clinical Practice, and is responsible for conducting an internal audit of the trial. The sponsor should agree with the investigator on the distribution of responsibilities (cf. 2.3 k).

2.2 Both the sponsor and investigator must agree on and sign the protocol as an agreement of the details of the clinical trial and the means of data recording (eg CRF). Any amendments to the protocol must have agreement of both sponsor and investigator before the amendment is implemented; any such agreement must be documented.

2.3 Particular responsibilities of the sponsor:

a) to select the investigator taking into account the appropriateness and availability of the trial site and facilities, and be assured of the investigator's qualifications and availability for the entire duration of the study; to assure the investigator's agreement to undertake the study as laid down in the protocol, according to these guidelines of Good Clinical Practice, including the acceptance of verification procedures, audit and inspection.

b) to inform the investigator of the chemical/pharmaceutical, toxicological, pharmacological and clinical information (including previous and on-going trials), which should be adequate to justify the nature, scale and duration of the trial, as a prerequisite to planning the trial and to inform the investigator of any relevant new information arising during the trial. All relevant information must be included in the Investigator's Brochure which must be supplemented and/or updated by the sponsor whenever new pertinent information is available.

c) to submit notification/application to the relevant authorities (when appropriate) and to ensure submission of any necessary documents to the Ethics Committee, and to ensure communication of any modification, amendment or violation of the protocol, if the change may impact on the subject's safety, and to inform the investigator and relevant authorities about discontinuation of the trial and the reasons for discontinuation.

d) to provide the fully characterized investigational medicinal product(s) prepared in accordance with Good Manufacturing Practice (GMP), suitably packaged and labelled in such way that any blinding procedure is ensured.
    Sufficient samples of each batch and a record of its analyses and characteristics must be kept for reference, so that there is the possibility for an independent laboratory to re-check the investigational products, eg for bioequivalence.

Records of the quantities of investigational medicinal products supplied must be maintained with batch/serial numbers. The sponsor must ensure that the investigator within his/her institution establishes a system for the safe handling, storage and use of the delivered investigational products (cf. 2.5 j).

e) to appoint, and ensure the on-going training of, suitable and appropriately trained monitors and their clinical research support personnel.

f) to appoint appropriate individuals and/or committees for the purpose of steering, supervision, data handling, statistical processing and trial report writing.

g) to consider promptly, jointly with investigator, all serious AEs and take appropriate measures necessary to safeguard trial subjects, and to report to appropriate authorities according to their requirements.

h) to inform promptly the investigator of any immediately relevant information that becomes available during a trial and ensure that the Ethics Committee is notified by the investigator(s) where required.

i) to ensure the preparation of a comprehensive Final Report of the trial suitable for regulatory purposes whether or not the trial has been completed. Safety up-dates may be required. For long-term trials an annual report may be required by the authorities.

j) to provide adequate compensation/treatment for subjects in the event of trial related injury or death, and provide indemnity (legal and financial cover) for the investigator, except for claims resulting from malpractice and/or negligence.

k) to agree with the investigator(s) on the allocation of responsibilities for data processing, statistical handling, reporting of the results, and publication policy.

MONITOR

2.4 The monitor is the principal communication link between the sponsor and the investigator.

Responsibilities of the monitor:

a) to work according to a predetermined SOP, visit the investigator before, during and after the trial to control adherence to the protocol and assure that all data are correctly and completely recorded and reported, and that informed consent is being obtained and recorded from all subjects prior to their participation in the trial.

b) to ensure that the trial site has adequate space, facilities (including laboratories), equipment, staff, and that an adequate number of trial subjects is likely to be available for the duration of the trial.

c) to ensure that all staff assisting the investigator in the trial have been adequately informed about and comply with the details of the trial.

d) to enable/ensure communication between the investigator and sponsor promptly at all times.

e) to check the CRF entries with the source documents and to inform the investigator of any errors/omissions.

f) to check that the storage, dispensing, return and documentation of the supply of investigational medicinal product(s) are safe and appropriate and in accordance with local regulations (cf. 2.5 j).

g) to assist the investigator in any necessary notification/application procedure.

h) to assist the investigator in reporting the trial data and results to the sponsor.

i) to submit a written report to the sponsor and the steering committee (if any) after each visit (monitor report) and after all relevant telephone calls, letters and other contacts with the investigator (audit paper trail concept).

INVESTIGATOR

2.5 Responsibilities of the investigator:

a) to be thoroughly familiar with the properties of the investigational medicinal product(s) as described in the Investigator's Brochure.

b) to ensure that he/she has sufficient time to conduct and complete the trial, and has adequate staff and appropriate facilities (including laboratories) which are available for the duration of the trial, and to ensure that other trials do not divert essential subjects or facilities away from the trial in hand.

c) to provide retrospective data on numbers of patients who would have satisfied the proposed entrance criteria during preceding time periods in order to assure an adequate recruitment rate for the trial.

d) to submit an up-to-date curriculum vitae and other credentials to the sponsor and — where required — to relevant authorities.

e) to agree and sign the protocol with the sponsor and confirm in writing that he/she has read, understands and will work according to the protocol and Good Clinical Practice, accepting the oversight of the monitor and control procedures, and agree with the sponsor on a publication policy.

f) to nominate (if appropriate) a local study coordinator to assist administration of the trial.

g) to submit notification/application to relevant bodies including local hospital management, and to the Ethics Committee, jointly with sponsor where appropriate.

h) to provide information to all staff members involved with the trial or with other elements of the patients' management.

i) to obtain informed consent from trial subjects prior to inclusion in the trial in accordance with principles described in sections 1.8 to 1.15.

j) to establish a system regarding investigational medicinal products to ensure that deliveries from the sponsor of such products are correctly received by a responsible person (eg a pharmacist); that such deliveries are recorded; that investigational products are handled and stored safely and properly; that investigational products are only dispensed to trial subjects in accordance with the protocol; that any unused products are returned to the sponsor. At the end of the trial, it must be possible to reconcile delivery records with those of usage and return stocks. Account must be given of any discrepancies. Certificates of delivery and returns must be signed.

k) to manage code procedures and documentation with meticulous care, and ensure that the treatment code is only broken in accordance with the protocol and that the monitor is consulted/informed when this is done.

l) to collect, record and report data properly.

m) to notify (with documentation) the sponsor and when applicable the Ethics Committee (and relevant authorities when required) immediately in the case of serious AEs and to take appropriate measures to safeguard subjects.

n) to make all data available to the sponsor/monitor and/or relevant authority (where required) for verification/audit/inspection purposes.

o) to sign and forward the data (CRFs), results and interpretations (analyses and reports) of the trial from his/her centre to the sponsor (and relevant authorities when required). Collaborative investigators and those responsible for the analyses (including statistical analyses) and the interpretation of the results should also sign.

p) to agree with and sign the Final Report of the trial. For multi-centre trials the signature of the coordinating investigator may suffice if agreed in the protocol.

q) to ensure that the confidentiality of all information about subjects is respected by all persons involved as well as the information supplied by the sponsor.

r) to observe the following points particularly related to patient care:
   - if appropriate, fully functional resuscitation equipment should be immediately available in case of emergency.
   - the investigator is medically responsible for those subjects who are under his/her care for the duration of the trial and must ensure that appropriate medical care is maintained after the trial.
   - clinically significant abnormal laboratory values or clinical observations must be followed up to the subject's benefit after completion of the trial.
   - subjects enrolled in a trial should be provided with a card bearing information identifying that he/she is in a trial if appropriate. Contact addresses/telephone numbers should be given in case of action needed at another place.
   - in the medical records it should be clearly marked that the subject is participating in a clinical trial.
   - the family doctor should normally, with the subject's consent, be informed.

Chapter 3: Data Handling

INVESTIGATOR

3.1   The investigator undertakes to ensure that the observations and findings are recorded correctly and completely in the CRFs and signed.

3.2   Entry to a computerized system is acceptable when controlled as recommended in the EC guide to GMP.

3.3   If trial data are entered directly into a computer there must always be adequate safeguard to ensure validation including a signed and dated print-out and back-up records. Computerized systems should be validated and a detailed description for their use be produced and kept up-to-date.

3.4   All corrections on a CRF and elsewhere in the hard copy raw data must be made in a way which does not obscure the original entry. The correct data must be inserted with the reason for the correction, dated and initialled by the investigator. For electronic data processing only authorized persons should be able to enter or modify data in the computer and there should be a record of changes and deletions.

3.5   If data are altered during processing, the alteration must be documented and the system validated.

3.6   Laboratory values with normal reference ranges should always be recorded on CRF or attached to it. Values outside a clinically accepted reference range or values that differ importantly from previous values must be evaluated and commented upon by the investigator.

3.7   Data other than those requested by the protocol may appear on the CRF clearly marked as additional findings, and their significance should be described by the investigator.

3.8   Units of measurement must always be stated, and transformation of units must always be indicated and documented.

3.9   The investigator should always make a confidential record to allow the unambiguous identification of each patient.

SPONSOR/MONITOR

3.10   The sponsor must use validated, error-free data processing programmes with adequate user documentation.

3.11 Appropriate measures should be taken by the monitor to avoid overlooking missing data or including logical inconsistencies. If a computer assigns missing values automatically, this should be made clear.

3.12 When electronic data handling systems or remote electronic data entry are employed, SOPs for such systems must be available. Such systems should be designed to allow correction after loading, and the correction must appear in an audit file (cf. 3.4 and 3.16).

3.13 The sponsor must ensure the greatest possible accuracy when transforming data. It should always be possible to compare the data print-out with the original observations and findings.

3.14 The sponsor must be able to identify all data entered pertaining to each subject by means of an unambiguous code (cf. 3.9).

3.15 If data are transformed during processing, the transformation must be documented and the method validated.

3.16 The sponsor must maintain a list of persons authorized to make corrections and protect access to the data by appropriate security systems.

ARCHIVING OF DATA

3.17 The investigator must arrange for the retention of the patient identification codes for at least 15 years after the completion or discontinuation of the trial. Patient files and other source data must be kept for the maximum period of time permitted by the hospital, institution or private practice, but not less than 15 years. The sponsor, or subsequent owner, must retain all other documentation pertaining to the trial for the lifetime of the product. Archived data may be held on microfiche or electronic record, provided that a back-up exists and that hard copy can be obtained from it if required.

3.18 The protocol, documentation, approvals and all other documents related to the trial, including certificates that satisfactory audit and inspection procedures have been carried out, must be retained by the sponsor in the Trial Master File.

3.19 Data on AEs must always be included in the Trial Master File.

3.20 The Final Report must be retained by the sponsor, or subsequent owner, for five years beyond the lifetime of his product. Any change of ownership of the data should be documented.

3.21 All data and comments should be made available if required by relevant authorities.

LANGUAGE

3.22 All written information and other materials to be used by patients and paraclinical staff must use language which is clearly understood.

3.23 Competent authorities have agreed to accept CRFs completed in English.

Chapter 4: Statistics

4.1 Access to biostatistical expertise is necessary before and throughout the entire trial procedure, commencing with designing of the protocol and ending with completion of the Final Report.

4.2 Where and by whom the statistical work shall be carried out should be agreed upon by both the sponsor and the investigator.

EXPERIMENTAL DESIGN

4.3 The scientific integrity of a clinical trial and the credibility of the data produced depend first on the design of the trial. In case of comparative trials the protocol should, therefore, describe:

a) an 'a priori' rationale for the target difference between treatments which the trial is being designed to detect, and the power to detect that difference, taking into account clinical and scientific information and professional judgement on the clinical significance of statistical differences;

b) measures taken to avoid bias, particularly methods of randomization when relevant.

RANDOMIZATION AND BLINDING

4.4 In case of randomization of subjects the procedure must be documented. Where a sealed code for each individual treatment has been supplied in a blinded, randomized study, it should be kept at the site of the investigation and with the sponsor.

4.5 In case of a blinded trial the protocol must state the conditions for which the code may/must be broken. A system is required enabling access to the treatment of individual subjects in case of an emergency. The system must only permit access to treatment key of one subject at a time. If the code is broken it must be justified in the CRF.

STATISTICAL ANALYSIS

4.6 The type(s) of statistical analyses to be used must be specified in the protocol, and any other subsequent deviations from this plan should be described and justified in the Final Report of the trial. The planning of the analysis and its subsequent execution must be carried out or confirmed by an identified, appropriately qualified and experienced statistician. The possibility and circumstances of interim analyses must also be specified in the protocol.

4.7 The investigator and monitor must ensure that the data are of high quality at the point of collection and the statistician must ensure the integrity of the data during their processing.

4.8 The results of analyses should be presented in a manner likely to facilitate the interpretation of their clinical importance, eg by estimates of the magnitude of the treatment effect/difference and confidence intervals, rather than sole reliance on significance testing.

4.9 An account must be made of missing and unused and spurious data during statistical analyses. All omissions of this type must be documented to enable review to be performed.

Chapter 5: Quality Assurance

5.1 A system of Quality Assurance, including all the elements described in this chapter and the relevant parts of the Glossary, must be employed and implemented by the sponsor.

5.2 All observations and findings should be verifiable. This is particularly important for the credibility of data and to assure that the conclusions presented are correctly derived from the raw data. Verification processes must, therefore, be specified and justified. Statistically controlled sampling may be an acceptable method of data verification in each trial.

5.3 Quality control must be applied to each stage of data handling to ensure that all data are reliable and have been processed correctly.

5.4 Sponsor audit must be conducted by persons/facilities independent of those responsible for the trial.

5.5 Any or all of the recommendations, requests or documents addressed in this Guideline may be subject to, and must be available for, an audit through the sponsor or a nominated independent organization and/or competent authorities (inspection).

5.6   Investigational sites, facilities and laboratories, and all data (including source data) and documentation must be available for inspection by competent authorities.

Annex

1. INTRODUCTION

This Annex is intended to provide guidance on some of the practical aspects of clinical trials. It includes much of the guidance contained in the 'Recommended Basis for the Conduct of Clinical Trials' (The Rules Governing Medicinal Products in the European Community, Vol. III. 1989, p. 115–132, Catalogue No. CB-55-89-843-EN-C, ISBN 92-825-9612-2). As parts of the guideline 'Recommended Basis for the Conduct of Clinical Trials' are now included in this Annex, the guideline will be revised accordingly.

2. GENERAL BACKGROUND

It is important for anyone preparing a trial of a medicinal product in humans that the specific problems of a particular clinical trial be thoroughly considered and that the chosen solutions be scientifically sound and ethically justified. It should be emphasized that this responsibility lies on the sponsor of a trial as well as on the actual investigator(s). Furthermore, considering the strategy of clinical evaluation of new active ingredients, it is highly advisable to plan and design the individual trial as a part of a logically constructed chain of investigations.

3. DEFINITION OF CLINICAL TRIALS

In this context, a clinical trial of medicinal product(s) means any systematic study in human subjects whether in patients or non-patient volunteers in order to discover or verify the effects of and/or identify any adverse reaction to the investigational products, and/or to study their absorption, distribution, metabolism and excretion in order to ascertain the efficacy and safety of the products.

   Clinical trials are generally classified into Phases I to IV. It is not possible to draw distinct lines between the phases, and diverging opinions about details and methodology do exist. Definitions (in brief) of the individual phases, based on their purposes related to clinical development of medicinal products, are given below.

a) Phase I:
   First trials of a new active ingredient in man, often healthy
   volunteers. The purpose is to establish a preliminary evaluation
   of safety and a first outline of the pharmacokinetic/dynamic
   profile of the active ingredient in humans.

b) Phase II:
   Therapeutic pilot studies. The purpose is to demonstrate
   activity and to assess short-term safety of the active ingredient
   in patients suffering from a disease or condition for which the
   active ingredient is intended. The trials are performed in a
   limited number of subjects and often, at a later stage, in a comparative (eg placebo-controlled) design. This phase also aims
   at the determination of appropriate dose ranges/regimens and
   (if possible) clarificiation of dose/response relationships, in
   order to provide an optimal background for the design of wider
   therapeutic trials.

c) Phase III:
   Trials in larger (and possibly varied) patient groups with the
   purpose of determining the short- and long-term safety/effi-
   cacy balance of formulations of the active ingredient, as well as
   to assess its overall and relative therapeutic value. The pattern
   and profile of more frequent adverse reactions must be investigated and special features of the product must be explored
   (eg clinically relevant drug interactions, factors leading to
   differences such as age etc). The design of trials should preferably be randomized double blind, but other designs may be
   acceptable for eg long-term safety studies. Generally the circumstances of the trials should be as close as possible to
   normal conditions of use.

d) Phase IV:
   Studies performed after marketing of the final medicinal
   product(s), although definition of this phase is not completely
   agreed upon. Trials in Phase IV are carried out on the basis
   of information in the summary of product characteristics of
   the marketing authorization, eg post-marketing surveillance,
   assessment of therapeutic value or strategies. According to
   the circumstances, Phase IV studies require trial conditions
   (including at least a protocol) such as described above for
   premarketing studies. After a product has been placed on the

market, clinical trials exploring, eg new indications, new methods of administration or new combinations, are considered as trials for new medicinal products.

4. MEASURES TO ENSURE OPTIMAL TRIAL CONDITIONS

A trial protocol (*see* item 6) must be worked out and adhered to, and proper instructions must be given to all involved.

The conditions of the physical framework in which the trial is carried out must be well arranged and carefully prepared. They must be of a sufficient quality, eg regarding supervision of patients/healthy volunteers, staffing, laboratory facilities (where necessary), emergency instructions, etc.

Finally, the distribution of responsibilities between the sponsor, the monitor and the investigator(s), and all collaborators must be clearly defined before the start of the clinical trial.

5. PRE-TRIAL DATA

Chemical, pharmaceutical, animal pharmacological and toxicological data on the substance and/or the pharmaceutical form in question must be available and professionaly evaluated before a new product is subjected to clinical trials. The sponsor's responsibility for providing exhaustive, complete and relevant material, eg by means of an Investigator's Brochure, is emphasized.

If an active ingredient is to be studied in Phase II, III and IV all existing research data in humans must be considered. Before Phase II studies are initiated, results from previous human pharmacology investigations are mandatory. Apart from effects on target functions, possible effects on other important organ systems should have been studied at relevant dosage levels, although it may not be possible in all studies. Results from kinetic studies of the active ingredient, its distribution and/or elimination, perhaps with several routes of administration, and results from other investigations on which the choice of dosage is based, eg studies of dose/response and/or concentration/effect relations and safety studies, must be considered. Before starting Phase III investigations, results from earlier clinical trials must be studied. The possibility of interactions with medicinal products containing other active ingredients should be given consideration.

6. TRIAL PROTOCOL

A well designed trial relies predominantly on a thoroughly considered, well structured and complete protocol. The protocol must, where relevant, contain the information given in the following list of items, or this list should at least be checked, whenever a trial is contemplated.

6.1   General information

    a)   title of the project

    b)   the name of the clinically responsible investigator(s) of the trial and the names of other possible participants and their professional background (eg 'medical doctor', 'biochemist', 'nurse', 'statistician', etc)

    c)   the name of the sponsor, if any

    d)   the clinic/department/group of physicians where the trial will take place (affiliations, addresses).

6.2   Justification and objectives

    a)   the aim of the trial

    b)   the reason for its execution

    c)   the essentials of the problem itself and its background, referring to relevant literature.

6.3   Ethics

    a)   general ethical consideration relating to the trial

    b)   description of how patients/healthy volunteers will be informed and consent will be obtained

    c)   possible reasons for not seeking informed consent.

6.4   General time schedule

    a)   description of the time schedules (including dates) of the trial, ie its start, investigation period and termination

    b)   justification of the time schedules, eg in the light of how far the safety of the active ingredients/medicinal products has been tested, the time course of the disease in question and expected duration of the treatment.

6.5   General design

    a)   specification of the type of trial, eg controlled study, pilot study, and preferably which phase it fits into

    b)   description of the randomization method, including procedure and practical arrangement

    c)   description of the trial design (eg parallel groups, cross-over design) and the blind technique selected (eg double blind, single blind)

    d)   specification of other bias reducing factors to be implemented.

6.6   Subject selection

a)   specification of the material (patients/healthy volunteers) including age, sex, ethnic groups, prognostic factors, etc where
relevant

b)   clear statement of diagnostic admission criteria

c)   exhaustive criteria for inclusion, pre-admission exclusions and
post-admission withdrawals of patients from the trial.

6.7   Treatment

a)   clear account of the product(s) to be used (marketing formulations, not 'laboratory drugs') and justification of the doses to
be used

b)   description of treatment applied to control group(s) or control
period(s) (placebo, other products, etc)

c)   route of administration, dose, dosing schedules, treatment
period(s) for the test product containing the active ingredient
and the comparative product(s)

d)   rules for the use of concomitant treatment

e)   measures to be implemented to ensure the safe handling of the
products

f)   measures to promote and control close adherence to the prescribed instructions (compliance monitoring).

6.8   Assessment of efficacy

a)   specification of the effect parameters to be used

b)   description of how effects are measured and recorded

c)   times and periods of effect recording

d)   description of special analyses and/or tests to be carried out
(pharmacokinetic, clinical, laboratory, radiological, etc)

6.9   Adverse events

a)   methods of recording adverse events

b)   provisions for dealing with complications

c)   information on where the trial code will be kept and how it can
be broken in the event of an emergency

d)   details for the reporting of adverse events, including by whom
and to whom it shall be done, and how fast the reports must
be submitted.

6.10   Practicalities

a)   a meticulous and specified plan for the various steps and
procedures in order to control and monitor the trial most
effectively

b) specifications and instructions for anticipated deviations from the protocol
c) allocation of duties and responsibilities within the research team and their coordination
d) instructions to staff, including trial description
e) addresses, telephone numbers, etc enabling any staff member to contact the research team at any hour
f) considerations of confidentiality problems, if any.

6.11 Handling of records

a) procedures for handling and processing records of effects and adverse events to the product(s) under study
b) procedures for the keeping of special patient lists and patient records for each individual taking part in the trial. Records should permit easy identification of the individual patient/healthy volunteer. A copy of the Case Report Form (CRF) should be included.

6.12 Evaluation

a) a specified account for how the response is to be evaluated
b) methods of computation and calculation of effects
c) description of how to deal with and report subjects withdrawn from/dropped out of the trial
d) quality control of methods and evaluation procedures.

6.13 Statistics

a) a thorough description of the statistical methods to be employed
b) the number of patients planned to be included. Reason for choice of sample size, including reflections on (or calculations of) the power of the trial and clinical justification
c) description of the statistical unit
d) the level of significance to be used
e) rules for the termination of the trial

6.14 Financing, reporting approvals, insurance, etc

In relation to the protocol it would often be advisable to state the attitude towards a series of problems, which directly or indirectly may influence performance and results of the trial.

The essentials are presented later in items 8–10 and include financing the trial, insurance and liability problems and labelling.

6.15 Summary, supplements

The protocol should comprise a comprehensive summary and relevant supplements (eg information to the patients, instructions to staff, description of special procedures).

6.16 References

A list of relevant literature, referred to in the protocol, must be included.

7. CASE REPORT FORMS

In order to adequately present the results of a clinical trial, it is essential that a fully comprehensive collection of information on the subject, the administration of the investigational medicinal product and the outcome of the protocol procedures is available. This is done using a Case Report Form (CRF) which should be established to facilitate observation of the subject, which also takes into account the protocol for the trial. In establishing a CRF, the following items should be considered. This list is not comprehensive and the CRF must take account of the nature of the investigational product. Omission of one or more of these items should be explained:

a) date, place and identification of the trial
b) identification of the subject
c) age, sex, height, weight and ethnic group of the subject
d) particular characteristics of the subject (eg smoking, special diet, pregnancy, previous treatment)
e) diagnosis; indication for which the medicinal product is administered in accordance with the protocol
f) adherence to the inclusion/exclusion criteria
g) duration of the disease; time to last break out (if applicable)
h) dose, dosage schedule and administration of the medicinal product; notes on compliance
i) duration of treatment
j) duration of the observational period
k) concomitant use of medicinal products and non-medicinal interventions/therapy
l) dietary regimens
m) recording of the effect parameters (including date, time, recorder's signature)
n) recorded adverse events. Type, duration, intensity, etc; consequences and measures taken
o) reason for withdrawal (if applicable) and/or breaking of the code.

8. FINANCING THE TRIAL

All financial problems involved in conducting and reporting a trial should be clearly arranged and a budget made out. Information should be available about the sources of economical support (eg foundations, private or public funds, sponsor/manufacturer). Likewise it should be clearly apparent how the expenditures are distributed, eg payment of volunteers, refunding expenses of the patients, payment for special tests, technical assistance, purchase of apparatus, possible fees to or reimbursement of the members of the research team, payment of the University/Clinic, etc.

Competent authorities may require detailed knowledge about the connection (economic etc) between the individual researcher and the manufacturer of the product(s) involved, in cases where such information is not obvious.

9. INSURANCE AND LIABILITY

Patients/healthy volunteers taking part in a clinical trial should be satisfactorily insured against any injury caused by the trial. The liability of the involved parties (investigators, sponsor/manufacturer, hospital/clinics, etc) must be clearly understood before the start of a trial of a medicinal product containing an active ingredient.

10. LABELLING

The provisions of Council Directive 65/65/EEC as amended on labelling should be applied by analogy to the labelling of medicinal products or placebo used in clinical trials. In addition, the labelling should include the words 'For clinical trial' and the name of the physician responsible for the trial (the investigator).

11. SYSTEMS OF NOTIFICATION/APPROVAL OF CLINICAL TRIALS

In Member States where regulation of medicinal products requires a notification or an application for approval before a trial is commenced the national rules must be consulted and complied with. In some countries a special form must be used. The notification/application must be signed by the investigator, the sponsor and the head of the institution or department where the trial is to take place. The person(s) signing will be held responsible for the performance of the trial, including all deviations from the protocol, in accordance with the national regulations. The notification/application usually should comprise the information specified in the form, a trial protocol with a brief summary and the information and documentation specified in the present document, but the requirements may vary among the Member States. For a product already authorized as a medicinal product, a reference to information previously submitted will usually be sufficient.

In general, notifications/applications should be filed with the competent authority in the following situations:

a) non-authorized products: all clinical trials
b) authorized medicinal products, if the trial is:
   - planned to explore new indications
   - carried out in patient groups not previously studied adequately
   - done with considerably higher dosages than previously approved.

Furthermore, Phase IV studies eg studies designed to determine the frequency of adverse reactions, or involving a very large number of patients to be treated (in accordance with the marketing authorization) for a very long period, or assessment of therapeutic strategies, may require to be notified.

A multi-centre trial (confined to one country) is in general to be regarded as one trial for which one complete notification/application with a master protocol and documentation should be submitted. In addition, each centre must submit a form confirming its participation in the trial.

Copied by permission of the Office for Official Publications of the European Communities.

Index